Data Interpretation in Critical Care Medicine

Commissioning Editor: Paul Fam
Project Development Manager: Claire Whittaker
Project Manager: Alan Nicholson
Design Manager: Andy Chapman

Data Interpretation in Critical Care Medicine

B. Venkatesh MBBS, MD(Int. Med), FFARCSI, FRCA, MD(UK), FJFICM
Associate Professor and Staff Specialist in Intensive Care
Royal Brisbane Hospital
University of Queensland
Australia

T. J. Morgan MBBS, FANZCA, FJFICM
Deputy Director and Senior Lecturer in Intensive Care
Mater Misericordiae Hospital,
University of Queensland
Australia

C. J. Joyce MB, ChB, FANZCA, FJFICM, PhD
Associate Professor and Senior Staff Specialist in Intensive Care
Princess Alexandra Hospital, University of Queensland
Australia

S. C. Townsend MBBS, FANZCA, FJFICM
Staff Specialist in Intensive Care
Royal Melbourne Hospital
Victoria, Australia

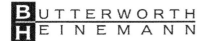
BUTTERWORTH
HEINEMANN

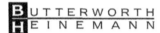

An imprint of Elsevier Science Limited

First published 2003

ISBN 075065273X

British Library Cataloguing in Publication Data
A catalogue record for this book is available from the British Library

Library of Congress Cataloging in Publication Data
A catalog record for this book is available from the Library of Congress

Note
Medical knowledge is constantly changing. As new information becomes
available, changes in treatment, procedures, equipment and the use of drugs
become necessary. The authors and the publishers have taken care to ensure
that the information given in this text is accurate and up to date. However,
readers are strongly advised to confirm that the information, especially with
regard to drug usage, complies with the latest legislation and standards of
practice.

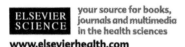

ELSEVIER
SCIENCE

your source for books,
journals and multimedia
in the health sciences

www.elsevierhealth.com

The
Publisher's
policy is to use
**paper manufactured
from sustainable forests**

Typeset by IMH(Cartrif), Loanhead, Scotland

Contents

Preface

The assessment of the ICU patient requires not only the powers of observation fundamental to the clinical examination of any patient, but also a thorough understanding of the information provided by 'numbers' generated from equipment and laboratory tests. In no other medical specialty is the correct interpretation of monitoring and laboratory data more important than in critical care medicine. This is reflected in the increasing emphasis on data interpretation in the qualifying examinations in intensive care. However, although a number of definitive texts on intensive care exist, few focus specifically on data interpretation in critical illness.

Accordingly, the ten chapters of this book are based around data sets that cover important systems. The format consists of brief clinical scenarios accompanied by a set of clinical, laboratory or radiological data, followed by a series of questions. The answers are provided at the end of each chapter with explanations. The pocket-book format makes it portable for access during 'breaks'. Whilst the data covered is not exhaustive, it rehearses the candidate in 'pattern recognition', an important element of training. Although the book is designed primarily for candidates preparing for the Australian Fellowship Examination in Intensive Care (FJFICM), it should be a useful resource for trainers and trainees in the specialty the world over.

We would like to thank our trainees, senior registrars and fellows in intensive care for keeping our minds ticking with their discussions, without which the stimulus for this book would not have arisen. Finally we would like to thank the staff of Elsevier Science for their assistance in the production of this book.

B. Venkatesh
T. J. Morgan
C. J. Joyce
S. C. Townsend

2002

1.

Blood gases

Question 1.1

You are called to the emergency department to review the blood gases of an obese 55-year-old hypertensive male who complains of daytime somnolence. He has the following arterial blood gas results:

Barometric pressure	760	mmHg
FiO_2	0.21	
Hb	190	g/L
pH	7.33	
PO_2	40	mmHg
PCO_2	64	mmHg
HCO_3-	33.3	mmol/L
Standard base excess	+5.4	mmol/L

A Describe the acid–base status.

B Calculate and interpret the A–a gradient.

C What is the likely diagnosis?

Question 1.2

You are called by a surgical resident medical officer (RMO) regarding the following blood gases, which were taken on a 73-year-old woman with chronic obstructive pulmonary disease admitted for work-up prior to elective cholecystectomy. The RMO requests advice on perioperative management of her chronic CO_2 retention and severe lung disease.

Barometric pressure	760	mmHg
FiO_2	0.21	
pH	7.55	
PO_2	63	mmHg
PCO_2	56	mmHg
HCO_3^-	48.3	mmol/L
Standard base excess	+22.7	mmol/L

A Why is she hypercapnic?

B Calculate and interpret her A–a gradient.

C Name three measures that can improve this kind of acid–base disturbance.

Question 1.3

You are asked to review a 15-year-old male who has been receiving treatment for asthma in the emergency department for 3 hours. The concern is persistent hypocapnia. He now is tachypnoeic with a mild generalized expiratory wheeze. The following are serial data from arterial blood.

Time	0700	1000
Barometric pressure	760 mmHg	
FiO_2	0.5	0.5
pH	7.5	7.39
PO_2	80	175 mmHg
PCO_2	30	30 mmHg
HCO_3^-	23.1	17.9 mmol/L
Standard base excess	-1.5	-7.9 mmol/L
Sodium	143	143 mmol/L
Chloride	105	105 mmol/L

A Calculate and interpret the respective A–a gradients.

B Describe the acid–base status at 0700 and at 1000 h.

C Has his asthma improved? Give reasons.

D What is the most likely explanation for the unchanging hypocapnia?

Question 1.4

A 20-year-old woman is involved in a motor vehicle accident. She is 32 weeks pregnant and has rib fractures, for which she has received analgesia. She is not shocked and her abdomen is non-tender. Her arterial blood gases and electrolytes are as follows:

Barometric pressure	760 mmHg
FiO_2	0.5
pH	7.32
PO_2	150 mmHg
PCO_2	42 mmHg
HCO_3^-	21.3 mmol/L
Standard base excess	−5.8 mmol/L

A Describe the acid–base status.

B Explain the acid–base status.

C Calculate and interpret the A–a gradient.

Question 1.5

A 45-year-old alcoholic woman treated with flucloxacillin for multiple staphylococcal lung abscesses has been improving, despite continuing pyrexia and muscle aches requiring regular oral paracetamol. After 3 weeks, while still in hospital, she becomes unwell again. Blood gas and biochemical data are as follows:

pH	7.21	
PCO_2	24 mmHg	
HCO_3^-	9.5 mmol/L	
Standard base excess	–18.4 mmol/L	
Sodium	135 mmol/L	(135–145)
Chloride	100 mmol/L	(100–110)
Creatinine	0.13 mmol/L	(0.07– 0.12)
Osmolar gap	8 mmol/kg	(<12)
Lactate	1.3 mmol/L	(<2.5)
β-Hydroxybutyrate	0.11 mmol/L	(<0.2)
D-Lactate and salicylate not detected		

A Give a general description of the acid–base disturbance.

B What is the likely diagnosis?

C What are the predisposing factors?

D How may the diagnosis be confirmed?

Question 1.6

An 18-year-old woman is suffering from acute renal failure owing to rhabdomyolysis post heroin overdose. She is haemodynamically stable and has been undergoing continuous venovenous haemodiafiltration with standard dialysis and replacement fluids for 8 days. The following are blood gas and biochemical measurements on an arterial blood specimen:

pH	7.455	
PCO_2	45 mmHg	
HCO_3^-	31.2 mmol/L	
Standard base excess	5.5 mmol/L	
Sodium	135 mmol/L	(135–145)
Potassium	3.2 mmol/L	(3.2–4.5)
Chloride	94 mmol/L	(100–110)
Lactate	5.0 mmol/L	(<2.5)
Albumin	22 g/L	(33–47)
Anion gap	10 mEq/L	

A Describe the acid–base status.

B Why is the anion gap not elevated in the presence of hyperlactaemia?

C What is the most likely explanation for the acid–base status?

Question 1.7

A 30-year-old man presents with fever, vomiting, sweatiness, confusion and agitation. The following values were measured on arterial blood:

FiO_2	0.21	
pH	7.4	
PO_2	105 mmHg	
PCO_2	25 mmHg	
HCO_3^-	15.3 mmol/L	
Standard base excess	−10.2 mmol/L	
Sodium	140 mmol/L	(133–145)
Chloride	105 mmol/L	(3.3–4.5)
Glucose	1.3 mmol/L	(3.0–7.8)

A Describe the acid–base status.

B Name two possible diagnoses.

Question 1.8

A 60-year-old woman presents with pneumonia, shock and respiratory distress. She has the following arterial blood gas results:

Barometric pressure	760 mmHg
FiO_2	0.5
pH	7.15
PO_2	105 mmHg
PCO_2	30 mmHg
HCO_3-	10.3 mmol/L
Standard base excess	−18.5 mmol/L

A Describe the acid–base status.

B Is there a problem with pulmonary oxygen transfer?

C Is intubation likely to be necessary?

Question 1.9

A prisoner is pulled unconscious from his cell after setting fire to his mattress. He has minor superficial surface burns. Blood gases and co-oximetry are as follows:

Barometric pressure	760 mmHg
FiO_2	0.4
Hb	15 g/dL
SaO_2	96%
pH	7.27
PO_2	60 mmHg
PCO_2	30 mmHg
HCO_3^-	13.6 mmol/L
Standard base excess	−13.7 mmol/L

A What are the acid–base abnormalities?

B Calculate and interpret the A–a gradient.

C Are there any other disturbances of oxygen transport?

D What are the likely diagnoses?

Question 1.10

The following are venous blood gas results from a man being treated for accelerated malignant hypertension.

FiO_2	0.21
pH	7.0
PO_2	75 mmHg
PCO_2	25 mmHg
HCO_3^-	6.1 mmol/L
Standard base excess	−24.7 mmol/L

A Describe the abnormalities.

B What is the likely mechanism?

C What action should be taken?

Question 1.11

You are asked to review the following blood gases of a patient receiving mechanical ventilation post laparotomy:

FiO_2	0.45
pH	7.27
PO_2	240 mmHg
PCO_2	75 mmHg
HCO_3-	34 mmol/L
Standard base excess	5.2 mmol/L

A Describe the acid–base status.

B Comment on the pulmonary oxygen transfer.

Question 1.12

A 40–year-old alcoholic woman became comatose with laboured breathing 18 hours after a drinking binge. Blood gases and electrolytes are set out below. Because the measured plasma lactate exceeded the reportable range for the bedside blood gas device (lactate oxidase method), it was also measured in the laboratory (lactate dehydrogenase method).

FiO_2	0.3	
pH	7.05	
PO_2	150 mmHg	
PCO_2	15 mmHg	
HCO_3^-	4.1 mmol/L	
Standard base excess	−25.8 mmol/L	
Sodium	135 mmol/L	(133–145)
Chloride	100 mmol/L	(98–108)
Lactate (lactate oxidase method)	>30 mmol/L	(<2.5)
Lactate (lactate dehydrogenase method)	3.9 mmol/L	(<2.5)

A What is the likely diagnosis?

B What simple laboratory tests are confirmatory?

C What treatment measures are indicated?

Question 1.13

Following a 6-hour debulking operation for ovarian malignancy, a patient is transferred to ICU. Blood biochemistry and arterial blood gas analysis on admission to ICU are as follows:

Sodium	145 mmol/L	(133–145)
Potassium	3.6 mmol/L	(3.3–4.5)
Chloride	120 mmol/L	(98–108)
pH	7.32	
PO_2	63 mmHg	
PCO_2	33 mmHg	
HCO_3^-	16.7 mmol/L	
Standard base excess	−10 mmol/L	

A Describe the acid–base status.

B What is the likely cause of this disturbance?

C What is the underlying biochemical mechanism?

Question 1.14

A patient presents with severe diabetic ketoacidosis. Eight hours after admission there is persistent acidaemia. Arterial blood gases and biochemical analysis are as follows:

Sodium	141 mmol/L	(133–145)
Potassium	3.6 mmol/L	(3.3–4.5)
Chloride	114 mmol/L	(98–108)
Glucose	10 mmol/L	(3.0–7.8)
pH	7.25	
PO_2	103 mmHg	
PCO_2	26 mmHg	
HCO_3^-	11.2 mmol/L	
Standard base excess	−16.2 mmol/L	

A Describe the acid–base abnormality.

B Is an increased dose of insulin required?

Question 1.15

You are called to the Emergency Medicine Department to review a 73-year-old man with mild abdominal pain who has a barrel chest and low saturations on pulse oximetry. A nurse hands you the following blood gas results, which were dictated to her over the telephone:

FiO_2	0.21
pH	7.34
PO_2	60 mmHg
PCO_2	60 mmHg
HCO_3^-	32 mmol/L
Standard base excess	-4.3 mmol/L
SaO_2	90%

A What is the pathophysiological mechanism of the hypoxia?

B Comment on the acid–base status.

Question 1.1: Answers

A Chronic respiratory acidosis with metabolic compensation.

B A–a gradient = 33 mmHg. This is above the normal upper limit when breathing air, even in elderly patients. Therefore the hypoxia is not purely due to hypoventilation – increased V/Q mismatch and/or shunt must also be operating.

C Obstructive sleep apnoea.

Question 1.2: Answers

A She has a severe primary metabolic alkalosis with appropriate respiratory compensation.

B A–a gradient = 20 mmHg. This is just above normal for an elderly person breathing air, suggesting that most of the hypoxaemia is due to hypoventilation.

C Correcting hypokalaemia, ceasing inciting agents such as diuretics, infusing saline, and possibly by administering parenteral acetazolamide.

Question 1.3: Answers

A A–a gradient has improved from 239 to 150 mmHg, indicating lessening V/Q mismatch and/or shunt.

B At 0700 h there was a primary acute respiratory alkalosis. At 1000 h this had changed to a dual acid–base disorder. There is now a respiratory alkalosis plus a metabolic acidosis with a raised anion gap (20 mEq/L).

C Yes. There is improving oxygenation and a lessening of the primary component of the respiratory alkalosis (but now there is a new element of respiratory compensation for a high anion gap metabolic acidosis).

D Salbutamol-induced lactic acidosis superimposed on improving bronchospasm.

Question 1.4: Answers

A Acute respiratory acidosis.

B At 32 weeks' pregnancy the normal $PaCO_2$ is 30 mmHg with compensatory HCO_3^- reduction. She now has acute CO_2 retention due to pain and narcotics, giving the appearance of an uncompensated metabolic acidosis. However, this must be interpreted in the light of the normal changes of pregnancy.

C Raised A–a gradient of 158 mmHg, suggesting shunt and/or $\dot{V}/\dot{Q}$ mismatch. Potential causes include further loss of FRC due to chest wall injury (already reduced by 500 mL in the third trimester), pulmonary contusions, pneumothorax.

Question 1.5: Answers

A Severe compensated metabolic acidosis with markedly raised anion gap (26 mEq/L).

B Pyroglutamic acidosis.

C Paracetamol and flucloxacillin administration in the setting of sepsis and renal and hepatic dysfunction.

D Urine screen for organic acids.

Question 1.6: Answers

A Compensated metabolic alkalosis, hyperlactaemia with normal anion gap.

B Hypoalbuminaemia reduces the sensitivity of the anion gap to unmeasured anions.

C Hyperlactaemia due to impaired metabolic conversion of lactate in the fluid used in renal replacement therapy (normal dialysate concentration 45 mmol/L). In this case, sufficient lactate has still been metabolized and replaced by HCO_3^- to produce a metabolic alkalosis.

Question 1.7: Answers

A The pH is normal in the setting of a severe respiratory alkalosis. This is therefore a mixed acid–base disorder due to a combination of a respiratory alkalosis and metabolic acidosis. The anion gap is raised, at 20 mEq/L.

B This acid–base disorder in combination with hypoglycaemia is seen in such conditions as salicylate poisoning (anion gap in this case due to salicylate and possibly lactate), fulminant hepatic failure with lactic acidosis, and septic shock.

Question 1.8: Answers

A The acidaemia is due to a mixed acid–base disorder, in this case a severe metabolic acidosis with coexisting respiratory acidosis.

B Yes. The A–a gradient is raised at 218 mmHg, implying shunt and/or $\dot{V}/\dot{Q}$ mismatch.

C Yes – she has an inappropriately high $PaCO_2$ for a metabolic acidosis. In the setting of shock and respiratory distress this indicates imminent respiratory muscle failure.

Question 1.9: Answers

A Metabolic acidosis with respiratory compensation.

B A–a gradient raised at 191 mmHg, implying V/Q mismatch and/or shunt.

C The combination of a high saturation at a PO_2 of 60 mmHg with acidaemia (which normally shifts the oxyhaemoglobin dissociation curve to the right) implies markedly increased haemoglobin–oxygen affinity.

D The likely diagnoses are inhalational injury, carbon monoxide poisoning (causing increased haemoglobin–oxygen affinity), lactic acidosis, possible cyanide poisoning.

Question 1.10: Answers

A Severe metabolic acidosis. Venous PCO_2 consistent with a degree of respiratory compensation. Elevated venous PO_2.

B Sodium nitroprusside-induced cyanide toxicity with cytochrome poisoning and lactic acidosis.

C Cease nitroprusside, administer antidote, e.g. cobalt ethylenediaminetetra-acetic acid (EDTA), sodium thiosulphate.

Question 1.11: Answers

A There is a partially compensated respiratory acidosis (at full compensation the expected $HCO_3^- = 37$ mmol/L. Alternatively, the expected standard base excess $= 12$ mmol/L).

B The A–a gradient is negative (−4.5 mmHg). Either the FiO_2 exceeded 0.45 at the time of sampling or there was a PO_2 measurement error.

Question 1.12: Answers

A Ethylene glycol poisoning – note the 'lactate gap' (the difference between the artefactually elevated lactate oxidase result and the lactate dehydrogenase method, which is free from interference) in the presence of a compensated high anion gap (31 mEq/L) metabolic acidosis.

B Osmolar gap. Urinalysis for oxalate crystals.

C Alcohol infusion, intravenous sodium HCO_3^-, urgent haemodialysis.

Question 1.13: Answers

A Normal anion gap metabolic acidosis with appropriate respiratory compensation.

B Large volume saline infusion causing 'dilutional' acidosis.

C Reduction of extracellular strong ion difference by large volume infusion with fluid with strong ion difference of zero.

Question 1.14: Answers

A Compensated metabolic acidosis, anion gap mildly elevated at 16 mEq/L.

B No, the anion gap is now only mildly elevated, indicating resolving ketoacidosis. The $\Delta AG : \Delta HCO_3^-$ ratio is approximately 3:13. Therefore the major proportion of the metabolic acidosis is hyperchloraemic, probably owing to saline extracellular fluid replenishment.

Question 1.15: Answers

A The patient has hypoxaemia, due mainly to hypoventilation. The A–a gradient is 18 mmHg, which is only mildly elevated for an elderly patient breathing air.

B There is a respiratory acidosis, with the degree of $[HCO_3^-]$ elevation being consistent with chronic compensated respiratory acidosis. An error has occurred when transcribing the SBE value: it has been written with the incorrect sign and should be + 4.3 mmol/L.

Calculations

A–a gradient

A–a gradient (mmHg) = $PAO_2 - PaO_2$ where PAO_2 is calculated from the alveolar gas equation:

$$PAO_2 = PiO_2 - (1 - FiO_2 \times (1 - R)) \times \frac{PaCO_2}{R}$$

$PaCO_2$ is arterial PCO_2. R is the respiratory exchange ratio, which is usually assumed to be 0.8. PiO_2 is calculated as $FiO_2 \times (BP - 47)$ where BP is barometric pressure and 47 is the saturated vapour pressure of water (mmHg). A simplified version of the alveolar gas equation in common use is:

$$PAO_2 = PiO_2 - \frac{PaCO_2}{0.8}$$

The normal A–a gradient ranges from 7 mmHg in young adults to 14 mmHg in elderly adults breathing air, and from 31 mmHg (young) to 56 mmHg (elderly) when breathing 100% oxygen.

$PaCO_2/[HCO_3^-]$ relationships in simple acid–base disturbances. $PaCO_2$ values are in mmHg, $[HCO_3^-]$ in mmol/L.

1. Acute respiratory acidosis.
   Expected $[HCO_3^-] = 24 + 0.1 \times (PaCO_2 - 40)$

2. Chronic respiratory acidosis.
   Expected $[HCO_3^-] = 24 + 0.35 \times (PaCO_2 - 40)$

3. Acute respiratory alkalosis.
   Expected $[HCO_3^-] = 24 - 0.2 \times (40 - PaCO_2)$

4. Chronic respiratory alkalosis.
   Expected $[HCO_3^-] = 24 - 0.5 \times (40 - PaCO_2)$

5. Metabolic acidosis.
   Expected $PaCO_2 = 1.5 \times [HCO_3^-] + 8$

6. Metabolic alkalosis.
   Expected $PaCO_2 = 40 + 0.6 \times [HCO_3^-]$

The four $PaCO_2$/SBE rules of simple acid–base disturbances (SBE in mmol/L, $PaCO_2$ in mmHg).

1. Acute respiratory acidosis and alkalosis $\Delta SBE = 0 \times \Delta PaCO_2$

2. Chronic respiratory acidosis and alkalosis $\Delta SBE = 0.4 \times \Delta PaCO_2$

3. Metabolic acidosis $\Delta PaCO_2 = \Delta SBE$

4. Metabolic alkalosis $\Delta PaCO_2 = 0.6 \times D\,SBE$

Anion gap

$$\text{Anion gap } (mEq/L) = [Na^+] - ([CL^-] + [HCO_3^-])$$

Further reading

Bia M, Their SO Mixed acid–base disturbances: a clinical approach. Med Clin North Am 1981; 65:347–361

Demling RH Smoke inhalation injury. New Horiz 1993; 1:422–434

Dempsey GA, Lyall HJ, Corke CF, Scheinkestel CD Pyroglutamic acidemia: a cause of high anion gap metabolic acidosis. Crit Care Med 2000; 28:1803–1807

Gin T, Ngan Kee WD Obstetric emergencies. In: Oh TE, ed. Intensive care manual. Oxford: Butterworth–Heinemann, 1997; 494–498

Iberti TJ, Leibowitz AB, Papadakos PJ, Fischer EP Low sensitivity of the anion gap as a screen to detect hyperlactaemia in critically ill patients. Crit Care Med 1990; 18:275–277

Kanber GJ, King FW, Eshchar YR, Sharp JT The alveolar–arterial oxygen gradient in young and elderly men during air and oxygen breathing. Am Rev Respir Dis 1968; 97:376–381

Maury E, Ioos V, Lepecq B, Guidet B, Offeenstadt G A paradoxical effect of bronchodilators. Chest 1997; 111:1766–1767

Morgan TJ, Hall JA Hyperlactaemia without acidosis – an investigation using an in vitro model. Crit Care Resusc 1999; 1:354–359

Morgan TJ, Venkatesh B, Hall J Crystalloid strong ion difference determines metabolic acid–base change during in vitro hemodilution. Crit Care Med 2002; 30:157–160

Narins RG, Emmett M Simple and mixed acid–base disorders: A practical approach. Medicine 1981; 59:161–187

Narins RG, Gardner LB Simple acid–base disturbances. Med Clin North Am 1980; 65:321–346

Nunn JF Distribution of pulmonary ventilation and perfusion. In: Nunn JF, ed. Applied respiratory physiology, 4th edn. Oxford: Butterworth–Heinemann, 1993; 156–197

Schlichtig R, Grogono AW, Severinghaus JW Human $PaCO_2$ and standard base excess compensation for acid–base imbalance. Crit Care Med 1998; 26:1173–1179

Venkatesh B, Morgan TJ, Garrett P The uses of error: measuring the lactate gap. Lancet 2001; 358:1806

Weekes JWN Poisoning and drug intoxication. In: Oh TE, ed. Intensive care manual. Oxford: Butterworth–Heinemann, 1997; 662–671

2

Biochemistry

Question 2.1

A 58-year-old man undergoes an uneventful thoracotomy and an oesophagectomy for carcinoma of the oesophagus. At operation a nasogastric tube and a feeding jejunostomy are placed. On day 4 in ICU the patient is difficult to wean off the ventilator.

Examine the plasma biochemistry:

	Pre–op	Day 4
Sodium	141 mmol/L	139 mmol/L (135–145)
Potassium	3.9 mmol/L	3.1 mmol/L (3.2–4.5)
Chloride	104 mmol/L	98 mmol/L (100–110)
Bicarbonate	26 mmol/L	28 mmol/L (22–33)
Glucose	5.2 mmol/L	6.8 mmol/L (3–7.8)
Phosphate	0.7 mmol/L	0.3 mmol/L (0.7–1.4)
Urea	3.6 mmol/L	2.8 mmol/L (3–8)
Creatinine	0.04 mmol/L	0.04 mmol/L (0.07–0.12)
Magnesium	0.7 mmol/L	0.6 mmol/L (0.7–1.0)

A What are the likely diagnoses for the above biochemistry?

B What is the most likely diagnosis?

Question 2.2

A previously well 24-year-old patient was admitted to ICU 4 hours after an elective arthroscopy with confusion and delirium.

Temp 39.2, HR 160/min, atrial fibrillation, BP 100/50

	Venous blood		
Sodium	145 mmol/L	(135–145)	
Potassium	3.7 mmol/L	(3.2–4.5)	**Coags**: NAD
Urea	8.3 mmol/L	(3–8)	
Creatinine	0.08 mmol/L	(0.07–0.12)	
AST	40 U/L	(<40)	
ALT	44 U/L	(<40)	
Glucose	8.6 mmol/L	(3–7.8)	
Hgb	145 g/L	(110–150)	
WBC	10.6×10^9/L	(4.0–11.0)	

A List three differential diagnoses.

B If the ionised Calcium (c) was 1.5 mmol/L (1.1–1.3), what is the likely diagnosis?

Question 2.3

A 36-year-old patient with abdominal pain and distension presented with the following biochemistry. He had had two admissions in the past year with similar complaints.

	Venous blood		Urea	8.5 mmol/L	(3–8)
Sodium	124 mmol/L (135–145)		Creatinine	0.09 mmol/L	(0.07 –0.12)
Potassium	4.5 mmol/L (3.2–4.5)		AST	40 U/L	(<40)
Chloride	104 mmol/L (100–110)		ALT	44 U/L	(<40)
Bicarbonate	18 mmol/L (22–33)		Alk phos	150 U/L	(40–110)
Calcium (c)	2.0 mmol/L (2.15–2.6)		LDH	550 U/L	(110–250)
Phosphate	1.1 mmol/L (0.7 –1.4)		Measured Osmolality	288 mosm/kg	(280–292)
Albumin	30 g/L	(33–47)	Glucose	8 mmol/L	(3–7.8)
Globulin	31 g/L	(25–45)	Lipase	2000 U/L	(<300)

A What is the most likely cause of his abdominal symptoms?

B What is the likely underlying aetiology of his abdominal condition?

C How will you manage this patient?

Question 2.4

A 34-year-old woman is admitted to ICU following a caesarean section for severe preeclampsia and fetal distress. She had been admitted to the labour ward 24 hours earlier for the management of preeclampsia. The case notes gave the following reasons for ICU admission:

Bradycardia, slow to wake up, poor cough, muscle weakness, hypotonic and hyporeflexic. Pupils equal and reactive to light.

Venous blood

Sodium	135 mmol/L	(135–145)
Potassium	3.8 mmol/L	(3.2–4.5)
Chloride	110 mmol/L	(100–110)
Bicarbonate	22 mmol/L	(22–33)
Urea	16.6 mmol/L	(3–8)
Creatinine	0.24 mmol/L	(0.07–0.12)
Coagulation screen	NAD	

A Suggest two possible diagnoses.

B Suggest two treatment measures for the likely diagnosis.

Question 2.5

Venous blood

Sodium	140 mmol/L	(135–145)
Potassium	2.5 mmol/L	(3.2–4.5)
Chloride	90 mmol/L	(100–110)
Bicarbonate	38 mmol/L	(22–33)
Urea	11.4 mmol/L	(3.0–8.0)
Creatinine	0.09 mmol/L	(0.07–0.12)
Total calcium	1.9 mol/L	(2.15–2.6)
Albumin	39 g/L	(33–47)

A Describe the electrolyte abnormalities.

B What is the underlying cause?

C List three aetiologies.

Question 2.6

Venous blood

Sodium	119 mmol/L	(135–145)
Potassium	6.8 mmol/L	(3.2–4.5)
Chloride	94 mmol/L	(100–110)
Bicarbonate	17 mmol/L	(22–33)
Glucose	2.6 mmol/L	(3.0–7.8)
Urea	14.8 mmol/L	(3.0–8.0)
Creatinine	0.13 mmol/L	(0.07–0.12)
Total calcium	2.74 mmol/L	(2.10–2.55)

A Describe the biochemical abnormalities.

B What is the likely diagnosis?

Question 2.7

Venous blood

Sodium	143 mmol/L	(135–145)
Potassium	4.1 mmol/L	(3.2–4.5)
Chloride	102 mmol/L	(100–110)
Bicarbonate	27 mmol/L	(22–33)
Urea	37 mmol/L	(3.0–8.0)
Creatinine	0.12 mmol/L	(0.07–0.12)

A What is the differential diagnosis of the above biochemistry?

Question 2.8

Venous blood

Sodium	133 mmol/L	(135–145)
Potassium	6.3 mmol/L	(3.2–4.5)
Chloride	106 mmol/L	(100–110)
Bicarbonate	21 mmol/L	(22–33)
Urea	13.0 mmol/L	(3.0–8.0)
Creatinine	0.28 mmol/L	(0.07–0.12)
Total calcium	1.85 mmol/L	(2.15–2.6)
Phosphate	2.69 mmol/L	(0.7–1.4)
Albumin	26 g/L	(33–47)
Globulins	35 g/L	(25–45)
Conjugated bilirubin	4 µmol/L	(1–4)
Total bilirubin	20 µmol/L	(4–20)
GGT	6 U/L	(0–50)
ALP	100 U/L	(40–110)
LDH	4020 U/L	(110–250)
AST	2130 U/L	(<40)
ALT	200 U/L	(<40)

A What are the biochemical abnormalities?

B What is the likely diagnosis?

Question 2.9

Venous blood

Sodium	130 mmol/L	(135–145)
Potassium	3.6 mmol/L	(3.2–4.5)
Chloride	102 mmol/L	(100–110)
Bicarbonate	25 mmol/L	(22–33)
Urea	12.6 mmol/L	(3.0–8.0)
Total protein	110 g/L	(62–83)
Albumin	32 g/L	(33–47)
Alk phos	92 U/L	(40–110)
Calcium	3.84 mmol/L	(2.15–2.6)
Phosphate	1.4 mmol/L	(0.7–1.4)

A What are the biochemical abnormalities?

B What is the likely diagnosis? How are the biochemical abnormalities explained?

Question 2.10

Arterial blood sample

pH	7.2	(7.36–7.44)
PCO_2	22 mmHg	(36–44)
PO_2	98 mmHg	(95–110)
Base excess	−16 mmol/L	(−2 to +2)
Bicarbonate	6 mmol/L	(22–33)
Sodium	138 mmol/L	(135–145)
Potassium	3.4 mmol/L	(3.2–4.5)
Chloride	110 mmol/L	(100–110)
Ionised calcium	0.96 mmol/L	(1.2–1.4)

A List six differential diagnoses for the above biochemistry.

Question 2.11

Arterial blood

pH	7.2	(7.36–7.44)
PCO_2	21 mmHg	(36–44)
PO_2	104 mmHg	(95–110)
Bicarbonate	7 mmol/L	(22–33)
Lactate	12 mmol/L	(< 2) mmol/L
Glucose	2.2 mmol/L	(3–7.8)

A List three differential diagnoses for the above biochemistry.

Question 2.12

A 64-year-old woman is brought to casualty in a confused state.

Arterial blood

pH	7.32	(7.36–7.44)
PCO_2	50 mmHg	(36–44)
PO_2	80 mmHg	(95–110)
Sodium	131 mmol/L	(135–145)
Potassium	4 mmol/L	(3.2–4.5)
Chloride	102 mmol/L	(100–110)
Bicarbonate	24 mmol/L	(22–33)
Glucose	2.4 mmol/L	(3–7.8)
CK	220 U/L	(50–150)
Cholesterol	8.4 mmol/L	(2.4 –6.2)

A What important diagnosis should be considered?

B List four treatment measures for this diagnosis.

Question 2.13

A previously well 40-year-old man suffered gunshot injuries to his abdomen, resulting in multiple bowel perforations which required surgical repair. He is now in the ICU and he is slow to wean off the ventilator. He is currently on TPN with the following formulation:

Total calories	3000
Proteins	70 g/day

An indirect calorimeter provided the following information:

VCO_2	400mL/min
VO_2	300mL/min

The arterial blood gases are as follows:

pH	7.35
PCO_2	54 mmHg
PO_2	70 mmHg
Base excess	+ 4.0 mmol/L

A Comment on the above data.

B Why is he slow to wean off the ventilator?

Question 2.14

A 53-year-old alcoholic is admitted to hospital after an alcoholic binge with a 1-day history of chest pain, vomiting and shortness of breath.

Chest X-ray	Left pleural effusion
Pleural fluid analysis	
pH	6.0
Cell count	800 cells/mm³
Protein	1 g/L
Amylase	800 U/L
Gram stain	Yeasts ++

A What is your diagnosis?

B How will you confirm your diagnosis?

Question 2.15

The following biochemistry was obtained from a patient who had undergone a therapeutic procedure in the intensive care unit.

Total protein	40 g/L	(60–80)
Albumin	25 g/L	(35–45)
Globulin	15 g/L	(25–30)
Antithrombin	0.3 U/mL	(0.7–1.3)
Protein C	0.3 U/mL	(0.5–1.3)
Plasma cholinesterase	3.6 kU/L	(4.1–8.8)
Ionized calcium	0.8 mmol/L	(1.1–1.3)

A Suggest an explanation for the above biochemistry.

Question 2.16

A 45-year-old man with Guillain–Barré syndrome is admitted to ICU. On day 4 of his illness he was noted to have the following plasma biochemistry:

Sodium	130 mmol/L	(135–145)
Potassium	3.6 mmol/L	(3.2–4.5)
Chloride	102 mmol/L	(100–110)
Bicarbonate	22 mmol/L	(22–33)
Urea	4 mmol/L	(3–8)
Glucose	4.2 mmol/L	(3–7.8)
Osmolality	290 mosm/kg	(280–292)
Total protein	100 g/L	(60–80)
Albumin	32 g/L	(35–50)
Alkaline phosphatase	92 U/L	(30–100)

A Comment on the above data.

Question 2.17

A previously fit 48-year-old patient was admitted with head injury to the ICU following an MVA. Seventy-two hours after admission he was noted to have the following biochemistry;

Venous blood

Sodium	131 mmol/L	(135–145)
Potassium	4.5 mmol/L	(3.2–4.5)
Urea	5.6 mmol/L	(3–8)
Creatinine	0.09 mmol/L	(0.07–0.12)
Glucose	6.8 mmol/L	(3–7.8)

Urinalysis

Urine micro	1 WCC, no red cells	
Urine sodium	60 mmol/L	(20–40)

A Give three differential diagnoses to explain the abnormal biochemistry.

Question 2.1: Answers

A

- Severe nasogastric losses
- Frusemide therapy
- Refeeding syndrome

B Refeeding syndrome.

The biochemical picture is one of hypokalaemic alkalosis.

In someone in whom feeding has been initiated, refeeding is associated with hypokalaemic, hypomagnesaemic and hypophosphataemic alkalosis. Profound hypophosphataemia is one of the cardinal features of the refeeding syndrome. The other common reason for this biochemical picture in the ICU include diuretic use and severe nasogastric losses. Frusemide therapy is unlikely to be the cause as urea is normally increased in patients on frusemide therapy because of prerenal azotemia. For the same reason, large fluid losses are unlikely to be the cause, unless there is concurrent volume replacement therapy. Other conditions presenting with hypokalaemic alkalosis include:

- Vomiting
- Villous adenoma of the rectum
- Steroid therapy, Cushing's syndrome and Conn's syndrome
- Laxative abuse.

Question 2.2: Answers

A The above combination of symptoms and signs raises a number of possibilities. The most likely ones are:

- Sepsis
- Malignant hyperpyrexia
- Thyroid storm.

B Thyroid storm. This is the typical picture of thyroid storm. However, sepsis will certainly need to be excluded

Other possibilities include hypoxia, hypercapnia and electrolyte abnormalities. Although these cause tachyarrhythmias and confusional states, the temperature is usually not elevated. In addition, such complications are uncommon in a fit young individual undergoing elective minor surgery. For the same reason sepsis is also unlikely. Also the normal FBC would argue against the diagnosis of sepsis. The normal levels of serum muscle enzymes and coagulation studies and the elevation of serum calcium concentrations would make the diagnosis of malignant hyperpyrexia unlikely. Although rare, postoperative delirium and fever should lead one to consider the diagnosis of thyroid storm, which may be the first presentation of thyrotoxicosis. Elevations in serum calcium levels in thyrotoxicosis result from increased osteoclast-mediated bone resorption.

Question 2.3: Answers

A The combination of abdominal pain, hypocalcaemia and hyperglycaemia would suggest the diagnosis of acute pancreatitis. The increase in serum urea reflects intravascular volume depletion.

B The most likely aetiology for the underlying condition is hyperlipidaemia. The clue to this is the presence of a pseudohyponatraemia (reduced serum sodium with normal measured serum osmolality). However, with the advent of ion-sensitive electrodes this is less of a problem.

C In addition to the conventional management of pancreatitis, plasmapheresis has been advocated for rapid reduction in serum triglyceride concentrations.

Question 2.4: Answers

A The two possible diagnoses are:

1. Incomplete reversal of neuromuscular blockade with neostigmine and inadequate dose of atropine

2. Hypermagnesaemia (which is the likely diagnosis).

Closer inspection of the biochemical data reveals an anion gap of 3. Anion gap is calculated as:

$$Na^+ - (Cl^- + HCO_3^-)$$

A reduced anion gap is seen with hypoalbuminaemia, hyperglobulinaemia, lithium intoxication, bromide intoxication, hypercalcaemia and hypermagnesaemia. Although there are reports of a low anion gap with hypermagnesaemia, subsequent published data suggest that if magnesium is administered as the sulphate salt, the anion gap may in fact be unchanged. Magnesium is used in the treatment of severe pre-eclampsia and target levels of 3–6 mmol/L are aimed for during therapy. Hypermagnesaemia is common in the setting of magnesium infusion and renal failure. The above clinical and laboratory features are consistent with hypermagnesaemia.

B Treatment measures include cessation of magnesium therapy, calcium administration (functional antagonist), diuretics and dialysis.

Question 2.5: Answers

A The abnormalities in the electrolyte profile are hypokalaemia, hypocalcaemia, hypochloraemia and an increase in plasma bicarbonate concentration.

B When hypokalaemia and hypocalcaemia coexist it is important to consider hypomagnesaemia. Magnesium is a cofactor for the enzyme Na–K ATPase in the renal tubules and hypomagnesaemia leads to a potassium loss in the urine. Hypocalcaemia in the setting of Mg deficiency results from a combination of deficient PTH secretion and inefficient PTH action on bone.

C The most common aetiologies for hypomagnesaemia include:

- Inadequate intake: Malnutrition, alcoholism

- Excessive losses: Diuretics, diarrhoea, drugs – amphotericin B, cisplatin

- Redistribution: Insulin administration, hungry bone syndrome.

Question 2.6: Answers

A The biochemical abnormalities are hyponatraemia, hyperkalaemia, hypoglycaemia, hypercalcaemia and azotaemia.

B These features are consistent with hypoadrenalism. The hyponatraemia is the result of hypocortisolaemia and increased levels of circulating ADH secondary to hypotension. The hyperkalaemia is secondary to reduced aldosterone. Hypoglycaemia and hypercalcaemia are also consistent with adrenal failure. Only 10–20% of patients with adrenal insufficiency develop hypercalcaemia. The aetiology of this is thought to be multifactorial: intravascular volume depletion, haemoconcentration of plasma proteins and the loss of antivitamin D effects of glucocorticoids. A combination of hyponatraemia and hyperkalaemia may be seen in renal failure. However, in this case the renal failure on its own is not severe enough to account for hyperkalaemia. Besides, hypoglycaemia is not common in renal failure. Spironolactone therapy can also result in hyponatraemia and hypokalaemia.

Question 2.7: Answer

A The results reveal an increased plasma urea and an associated increase in urea:creatinine ratio. The normal level is 50–100:1. A disproportionate increase in urea over creatinine could be due to:

- dehydration (excretion of urea is dependent not only on GFR, but also on the urine flow rate). In dehydration leading to progressive reduction in GFR, urine flow rate decreases, resulting in increased urea reabsorption in the distal tubules, thereby giving rise to increased urea:creatinine ratios

- High-protein meal

- GI bleed (resulting in increased protein delivery into the GI tract)

- Steroid therapy.

Question 2.8: Answers

A The abnormalities include hyperkalaemia, hypocalcaemia, hyperphosphataemia, elevations in urea and creatinine with a low urea:creatinine ratio, and significant elevations in AST and LDH with minor increase in ALT.

B The likely diagnosis is rhabdomyolysis. The triad of hyperkalaemia, hyperphosphataemia and hypocalcaemia suggest cell breakdown, which may be seen in tumour lysis syndrome and rhabdomyolysis.

A low urea:creatinine ratio is seen in rhabdomyolysis (excess production of creatinine from muscle) and diabetic ketoacidosis (acetoacetate interferes with Jaffe's picric acid method of estimating creatinine). The increase of serum enzymes – mainly AST and LDH as compared to ALT – suggests that the enzymes arise from muscle damage. (ALT is more liver specific, but is also in kidneys – AST more widespread – in RBC, muscle etc.).

Question 2.9: Answers

A The biochemical abnormalities are hyponatraemia, hypercalcaemia, hyperglobulinaemia and reduced anion gap.

B The combination of hyperglobulinaemia, hypercalcaemia and a normal alkaline phosphatase suggests the diagnosis of multiple myeloma. The low anion gap is the result of a net positive charge from cationic paraproteins resulting in increased urinary Cl⁻ reabsorption to maintain electroneutrality. The hyponatraemia is factitious, resulting from hyperproteinaemia.

Question 2.10: Answer

A Causes of metabolic acidosis with ionized hypocalcaemia include:

1. Acute pancreatitis (acidosis, usually lactic, due to hypotension, hypoxia, and tissue hypoperfusion, hypocalcaemia due to calcium precipitation). Lipase levels may be diagnostic.

2. Tumour lysis syndrome (acidosis due to lactate, sulphates, phosphates and urates released from necrotic tumour cells, and hypocalcaemia secondary to the hyperphosphataemia). History and biochemistry diagnostic.

3. Rhabdomyolysis (pathogenesis of acidosis and hypocalcaemia similar to tumour lysis syndrome). Raised CK and elevated creatinine:urea ratio are diagnostic.

4. Acute renal failure (although the degree of acidosis seen above is uncommon in acute renal failure).

5. Ethylene glycol intoxication (high anion gap acidosis due to lactate, oxalate and glycolate and hypocalcaemia secondary to Ca oxalate excretion in the urine). Elevated osmolar gap and presence of crystalluria diagnostic.

6. Hydrofluoric acid intoxication (acidosis due to fluoride, low calcium due to precipitation in soft tissue). Presence of burns is diagnostic.

Question 2.11: Answer

A

- Liver disease
- Seizures
- Alcohol intoxication.

The biochemical data reveal hypoglycaemia and metabolic acidosis with a raised lactate. These three conditions produce a combination of hypoglycaemia and a lactic acidosis. Metformin produces a lactic acidosis but usually does not cause hypoglycaemia in standard doses. However, in overdose, or during a severe metformin-induced acidosis, hypoglycaemia may occur. An example of this is given in the case report by Kruse et al (see Further reading).

Question 2.12: Answers

A Myxoedema coma. The combination of hyponatraemia, hypoglycaemia and hypercholesterolaemia is highly suggestive of myxoedema coma. Although this is an uncommon entity, biochemical patterns may be useful in pointing to the diagnosis, which can be confirmed by thyroid function tests.

B

- Intravenous T_3 or T_4

- Intravenous fluids

- Rewarming

- As there is a risk of coexisting adrenal insufficiency or precipitation of the same, when thyroxine treatment is commenced, steroids are recommended as part of the initial management.

Question 2.13: Answers

A This patient is being overfed. The caloric requirements of this patient can be derived using the Weir equation.

$$\text{Energy expenditure} = \frac{[3.9 \text{ VO}_2 \text{ mL/min} + 1.1 \text{ VCO}_2 \text{ mL/min}]}{-2.2 \text{ urinary nitrogen g/day}}.$$

In practice, the amount of urinary nitrogen is not measured as its contribution to energy expenditure is minimal. The respiratory quotient is over 1. This suggests that the patient is either acutely hyperventilated, or there is overfeeding.

B The caloric requirement based on this patient's indirect calorimetry data amounts to approximately 1600 Kcal/day. Any excess calories will be converted to fat. The process of conversion of carbohydrate to fat has an RQ of 8, owing to excess CO_2 production. Hence the inability to wean off the ventilator rapidly.

Question 2.14: Answers

A Boerhaave's syndrome – perforated oesophagus. Although the chest pain and a high amylase concentration in the pleural fluid would lead one to suspect a pancreatitis-related pleural effusion, the presence of yeasts in the pleural fluid is highly suggestive of a perforated oesophagus. An elevated amylase concentration is also in keeping with this (salivary source of amylase).

B Gastrografin swallow.

Question 2.15: Answer

A The history and results are consistent with a patient who has undergone plasmapheresis. There is a general reduction in all plasma protein concentrations. The hypocalcaemia is due to the chelation of calcium by citrate used as an anticoagulant.

Liver disease might produce a general reduction in plasma protein concentrations, but hypocalcaemia is unlikely.

Question 2.16: Answer

A The results are consistent with a pseudohyponatraemia (hyponatraemia, normal measured serum osmolality and a raised osmolar gap of 22). This is due to the administration of γ-globulin for the therapy of Guillain–Barré syndrome.

Pseudohyponatraemia is seen in the setting of hyperlipidaemia or hyperproteinaemia.

SIADH is also seen in these patients, but it is normally accompanied by a reduction in measured serum osmolality.

Question 2.17: Answers

A The three likely differential diagnoses in this setting are:

• SIADH (Syndrome of Inappropriate ADH secretion)

• Cerebral salt wasting

• Inappropriate use of hypotonic IV solutions.

SIADH is frequently seen after head injury and is diagnosed on the basis of a low serum sodium and a high urine sodium concentration in the absence of renal, adrenal or thyroid dysfunction. Cerebral salt wasting (CSW) syndrome is an entity which bears a number of similarities to SIADH. The main differentiating point between CSW and SIADH is thought to be the presence of volume depletion and polyuria in the former. Although some investigators question the existence of this syndrome, others believe it is important to distinguish between the two. The biochemical criteria used for distinguishing between fluid-replete and fluid-depleted states, such as raised serum urea, urate and ADH levels, have not been shown to be reliable. The treatment for SIADH is fluid restriction, whereas fluid repletion would be the mainstay of management for CSW. Inappropriate use of hypotonic IV fluids will result in a low serum and urine sodium concentration.

Further reading

Akmal M, Bishop JE, Telfer N, Norman AW, Massry SG Hypocalcemia and hypercalcemia in patients with rhabdomyolysis with and without acute renal failure. J Clin Endocrinol Metab 1986; 63:137–142

Dacey M Hypomagnesemic disorders. Crit Care Clin 2001; 17:155–173

DeMartino GN, Goldberg AL A possible explanation of myxedema and hypercholesterolemia in hypothyroidism: control of lysosomal hyaluronidase and cholesterol esterase by thyroid hormones. Enzyme 1981; 26:1–7

Dunn CJ, Peters DH Metformin. A review of its pharmacological properties and therapeutic use in non-insulin-dependent diabetes mellitus. Drugs 1995; 49:721–749

Emmett M, Narins RG Clinical use of the anion gap. Medicine (Baltimore) 1977; 5:38–54

Hierholzer K, Finke R. Myxedema Kidney Int 1997; 59 (Suppl):S82–89

Houston MC Pleural fluid pH: diagnostic, therapeutic, and prognostic value. Am J Surg 1987; 154:333–337

Howard JM, Reed J Pseudohyponatremia in acute hyperlipemic pancreatitis. A potential pitfall in therapy. Arch Surg 1985; 120:1053–1055

Kruse JA Metformin-associated lactic acidosis. J Emerg Med 2001; 20:267–272

Lawn N, Wijdicks EF, Burritt MF Intravenous immune globulin and pseudohyponatremia. N Engl J Med 1998; 339:632

Lennertz A, Parhofer KG, Samtleben W, Bosch T Therapeutic plasma exchange in patients with chylomicronemia syndrome complicated by acute pancreatitis. Ther Apher 1999; 3:227–233

Luft FC Lactic acidosis update for critical care clinicians. J Am Soc Nephrol 2001; 12(Suppl 17):S15–19

Maesaka JK, Gupta S, Fishbane S Cerebral salt-wasting syndrome: does it exist? Nephron 1999; 82(2):100–109

Marik PE, Bedigian MK Refeeding hypophosphatemia in critically ill patients in an intensive care unit. A prospective study. Arch Surg 1996; 131: 1043–1047

Miell J, Wassif W, McGregor A, Butler J, Ross R Life–threatening hypercalcaemia in association with Addisonian crisis. Postgrad Med J 1991; 67:770–772

Morisaki H, Yamamoto S, Morita Y, Kotake Y, Ochiai R, Takeda J Hypermagnesemia-induced cardiopulmonary arrest before induction of anesthesia for emergency cesarean section. J Clin Anesth 2000; 12:224–226

Pain RW. Test and teach. Number forty–one. Diagnosis: hypertriglyceridemia with pseudohyponatremia in acute or chronic alcoholism; multiple myeloma with pseudohyponatremia, decreased anion gap and hypercalcemia. Pathology 1983; 15:233, 331–334

Prasad VM, Erickson R, Contreras ED, Panelli F Spontaneous candida mediastinitis diagnosed by endoscopic ultrasound-guided, fine-needle aspiration. Am J Gastroenterol 2000; 95:1072–1075

Ringel MD. Management of hypothyroidism and hyperthyroidism in the intensive care unit. Crit Care Clin 2001; 17:59–74

Sherr HP, Light RW, Merson MH, Wolf RO, Taylor LL, Hendrix TR Origin of pleural fluid amylase in esophageal rupture. Ann Intern Med 1972; 76:985–986

Silverstein FJ, Oster JR, Materson BJ et al. The effects of administration of lithium salts and magnesium sulfate on the serum anion gap. Am J Kidney Dis 1989; 13:377–381

Solomon SM, Kirby DF. The refeeding syndrome: a review. JPEN J Parent Enteral Nutr 1990; 14:90–97

Vasikaran SD, Tallis GA, Braund WJ Secondary hypoadrenalism presenting with hypercalcaemia. Clin Endocrinol (Oxf) 1994; 41:261–264

Vaswani SK, Sprague R Pseudohyponatremia in multiple myeloma. South Med J 1993; 86:251–252

Zaloga G, Marik PE Hypothalamic–pituitary–adrenal disorders. Crit Care Clin 2001; 17:25–42

Zaloga GP Hypocalcemia in critically ill patients. Crit Care Med 1992; 20:251–262

3.

Cardiovascular

Question 3.1

Aortic pressure wave trace of a 55-year-old man 12 hours post CABG with an intra-aortic ballon pump (IABP) in situ. He has cold peripheries, BP 90/45, is oliguric, and has developed a lactic acidosis.

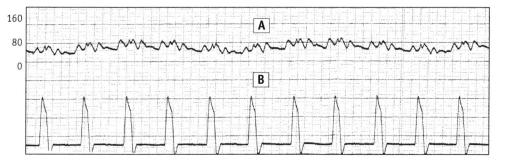

Curve A is aortic pressure trace. Curve B is balloon pressure trace.

A Describe the IABP trace.

B Assuming a normal preload, from the trace, what single measure could be employed to improve his circulation?

Question 3.2

ECG of a 44-year-old woman presenting with shortness of breath.

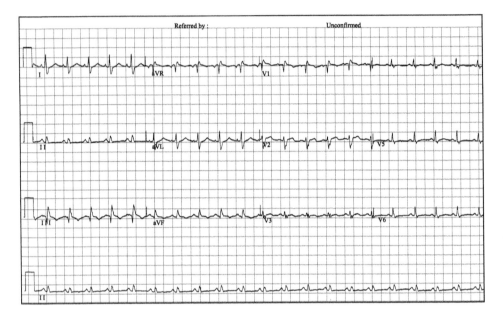

A Suggest a likely diagnosis.

Question 3.3

An ECG recorded from a 3-year-old child.

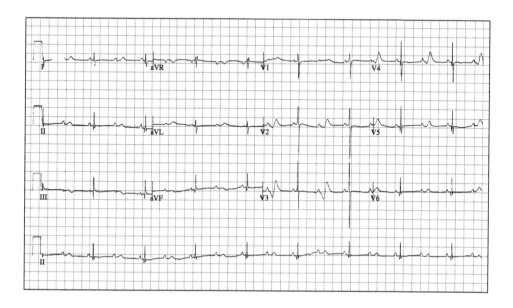

A Analyse the ECG.

Question 3.4

ECG recorded after resuscitation in a 55-year-old man who suffered an out-of-hospital cardiac arrest.

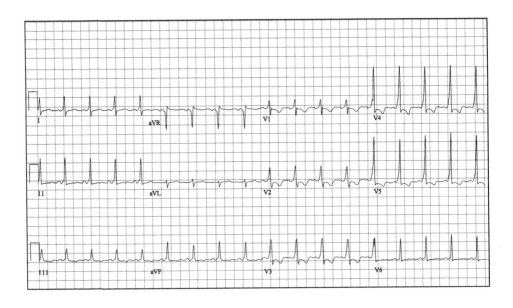

A Analyse the ECG.

Question 3.5

ECG taken from a 77-year-old woman presenting with dyspnoea.

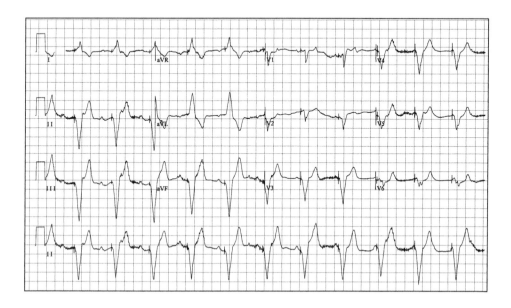

A Analyse the ECG and comment on the abnormalities.

Question 3.6

A 30-year-old man presents after a high-speed motorbike accident.

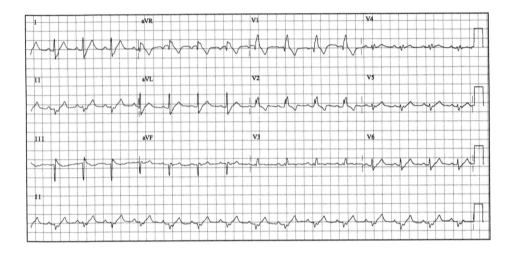

A Examine the ECG and comment on relevant findings.

Question 3.7

Examine the following ECG taken from a 65-year-old man with chest pain.

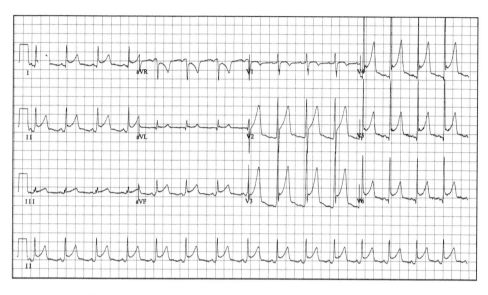

A What is the likely cause of his symptoms?

Question 3.8

Examine the following ECG taken from a 65-year-old woman.

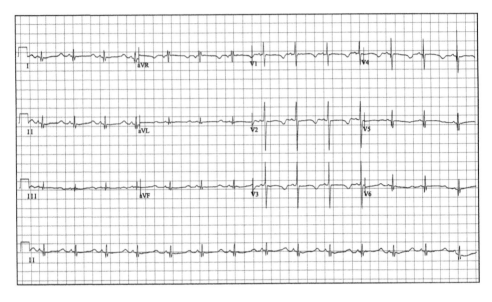

A Comment on the findings.

Question 3.9

Examine the ECG taken from a 48-year-old woman presenting with chest pain and hypotension.

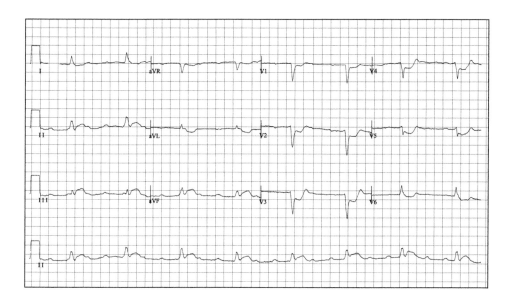

A Comment on the findings.

Question 3.10

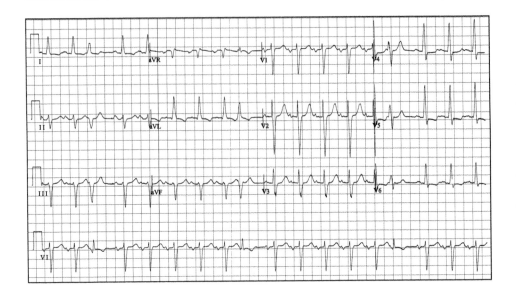

Examine this ECG.

A Comment on the findings.

Question 3.11

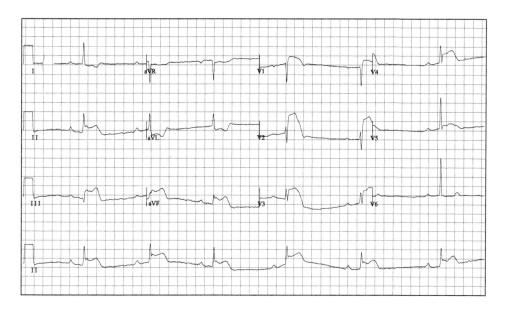

Examine this ECG and comment on the findings.

Question 3.12

A 47-year-old 90 kg man presents in shock after a large LAD territory myocardial infarct (MI). He is ventilated FiO$_2$ 0.5 and PEEP 5 cmH$_2$O. He has been heparinized and is receiving dopamine at 4.4 μg/kg/min and dobutamine at 5.5 μg/kg/min. He is tachycardic, HR 125 and BP 76/ 65, and an intra-aortic balloon pump is in situ. His pulmonary artery catheter data are as follows:

CVP	18 mmHg	(0–8)
PA	31/20 mmHg	(25/9)
PAOP	19 mmHg	(6–12)
CI	1.8 L/m/m²	(≥2.5)
SVRI	2311 dynes/s/cm^{-5}/m²	(1800–2200)
PVR	155 dynes/s/cm^{-5}	(120–250)
Temp.	38.4 °C	

A Suggest a possible diagnosis for the above set of data.

B What other tests might support your diagnosis?

C Suggest further management.

Question 3.13

A 58-year-old woman with a history of hypertension and moderate aortic stenosis is scheduled for an aortic valve replacement. Postoperatively her course is complicated by hypotensive episodes and a late systolic murmur is auscultated over the precordium. An echocardiograph demonstrates the following findings:

Transoesophageal echocardiograph report:

Vigorous LV function with no RWMAs and LVEF 60%. Marked LV hypertrophy. RV function normal. Aortic valve prosthesis shows no evidence of regurgitation or stenosis. Left ventricular outflow tract shows a reduced cross-sectional area during systole, with obliteration of the chamber cavity and an estimated peak gradient of 65 mmHg. Trivial mitral regurgitation. No evidence of pericardial effusion or clot.

A What is the cause of this patient's haemodynamic instability and how would you proceed with treatment?

Question 3.14

A 45-year-old man presents with staphylococcal endocarditis involving the mitral valve. He undergoes surgical debridement and replacement of the valve with a mechanical prosthesis. One week later his blood count is as follows:

Hb	85 g/L	(135–180)
MCV	92 fL	(80–98)
WBC	12.5 × 10⁹/L	(4.0–11.0)
Neutrophils	8.4 × 10⁹/L	(2.00–8.00)
Platelets	35 × 10⁹/L	(140–400)
Platelet Factor IV	IgG positive	

Blood film shows evidence of schistocytes, reticulocytes, toxic granulation of white cells and reduced platelet numbers with some large basophilic platelets.

Clinically he remains septic, with mild splenomegaly, a petechial rash and a pansystolic murmur audible at the apex.

A Give a differential diagnosis for the observed thrombocytopenia.

Question 3.15

A 78-year-old 70 kg man presents with chest pain and ECG changes consistent with an acute anteroseptal infarct. He is noted to be hypotensive and a pulmonary artery flotation catheter is inserted to guide his resuscitation. His haemodynamic and blood gas data are as follows:

HR	145 bpm	
MAP	55 mmHg	
CVP	10 mmHg	(0–8)
SVO_2 (PA)	85%	(75% approx.)
PAP	26 mmHg	(25/9)
CI	1.6 L/m/m$_2$	($\geq$2.5)
PAOP	18 mmHg	(6–12)
SVRI	2250 dynes/s/cm^{-5}/m^2	(1800–2200)
FiO_2	0.6	
pH	7.28	
$PaCO_2$	38 mmHg	
PaO_2	115 mmHg	
SaO_2	99%	

A Interpret the data.

Question 3.16

A 40-year-old woman is referred for assessment of poor exercise tolerance. Her ECG and cardiac catheterization data are as follows:

ECG shows sinus rhythm, tall R waves in V1 with RAD, P pulmonale and TWI V1–4.

Aortic BP	140/100 mmHg	(130/80)
RA(mean)	16 mmHg	(0–6)
RV	91/16 mmHg	(25/0–6)
PA	92/40/60 mmHg	(25/6–12)
PAOP	6 mmHg	(6–12)
PAO$_2$	61%	(75% approx.)
Arterial SO$_2$	97%	
CI	1.8 L/m/m²	(≥2.5)

A Interpret the ECG and haemodynamic data. What is the likely cause of this patient's symptoms?

You are asked to perform a nitric oxide provocation test in the intensive care unit. The data obtained are as follows:

	FiO$_2$	SaO$_2$(%)	Inspired nitric oxide (ppm)	PA (mmHg)
Time				
1600	0.21	96	0	78/37/52
1605	1.0	100	0	71/31/48
1610	1.0	100	14	64/27/41
1615	1.0	100	38	62/22/39
1620	1.0	100	0	75/32/47

B Interpret the results and explain the relevance of these findings.

Question 3.17

Swan–Ganz data obtained from a 42-year-old woman weighing 116 kg ventilated on 40% oxygen, mean airway pressure 20 cmH$_2$O and PEEP 12 cmH$_2$O. Inotropic support dopamine 5 μg/kg/m and noradrenaline (norepinephrine) 0.04 μg/kg/m. Temperature 38.5°C.

Time	1200	1230
Nitric oxide	0	20 ppm
FiO$_2$	0.4	0.4
HR	81	82 bpm
MAP	81	85 mmHg
CVP	22	21 mmHg
PAOP	21	21 mmHg
PAS	60	56 mmHg
PAM	49	44 mmHg
PAD	44	38 mmHg
CO	10.7	12.1 L/m (thermodilution method)
CI	4.9	5.5 L/m/m^2
CO	7.5	8.9 L/m (oesophageal Doppler method)
SVRI	969	930 dynes/s/cm^{-5}/m^2
PVRI	460	334 dynes/s/cm^{-5}

A Interpret the haemodynamic data.

B Suggest a possible cardiac lesion and give evidence.

C What is the explanation for the measured high cardiac output?

Question 3.1: Answers

A The trace reveals a 1:2 timing. Increase augmentation of IABP; the diastolic augmented pressure is equal to systolic pressure in the trace.

B 1:1 timing of IABP; the balloon inflation is currently set at 1:2 timing.

The following criteria are used to ensure optimum timing of an IABP in situ:

- The inflation occurs at the dicrotic notch.
- The slope of the rise of the augmented diastolic waveform is straight and parallel to the systolic upstroke.
- The augmented diastolic pressure should exceed or at least equal end-systolic pressure.
- The end-diastolic pressure at balloon deflation is lower than the preceding unassisted end-diastolic pressure by 15–20 mmHg.
- The systolic pressure following a cycle of balloon inflation (assisted systolic pressure) is lower than the previous unassisted systolic pressure by about 5 mmHg.

The efficiency of a balloon pump is affected by:

- Timing of inflation and deflation
- Assist ratio
- Heart rate (tachycardia >130-140 reduces the benefit from a balloon pump)
- Gas loss from the balloon
- A minimum cardiac index of 1.2–1.4 L/min/m^2 is required for an IABP to be effective.

Question 3.2: Answer

A A diagnosis of pulmonary embolism is supported by tachycardia with a SI, QIII, T III pattern.

The ECG findings of pulmonary embolism (PE) are most likely related to acute pulmonary hypertension, right atrial and ventricular dilatation, hypoxia and myocardial ischaemia. It is important to note that ECG findings are not diagnostic but only suggestive of PE. The most common ECG finding in PE is sinus tachycardia. An ECG diagnosis of PE is considered when three or more of the following signs are present:

- Incomplete or complete RBBB pattern (due to abrupt stretch of the right fascicle of His)
- S waves in lead I and aVL (>1.5 mm)

- Clockwise rotation
- Q waves in lead III and aVF
- Right axis or an indeterminate axis
- Inverted T waves in leads III and aVF
- Atrial arrhythmias (due to atrial dilatation).

Question 3.3: Answer

A

- Bradycardia HR ~50 bpm
- Second-degree heart block with 1:2 conduction
- Prolonged QT interval ~680 ms.

The commonest cause of heart block in children is congenital, although connective tissue diseases in the mother may predispose to heart block in the child. Prolongation of the QT interval may be a consequence of the bradycardia. However, other causes must be considered: Hypokalaemia, hypomagnesaemia and drugs (quinidine, procainamide).

Question 3.4: Answer

A Wolff–Parkinson–White syndrome type A, as evidenced by the presence of δ waves, widened QRS complex, shortened PR interval and dominant R wave in V1 and V2.

Other pre-excitation syndromes include:

- Lown–Ganong–Levine syndrome (characterized only by a short PR interval)
- Syndromes related to atrio-Hisian tracts
- Syndromes related to nodoventricular fibres (fibres of Mahaim).

Question 3.5: Answer

A Third-degree heart block with P waves dissociated from the QRS complex, pacing spikes, left axis deviation and widening of the QRS complex. The paced rate is approximately 70 bpm.

Question 3.6: Answer

A Right bundle branch block with an associated left axis, suggestive of left anterior fascicle block. A myocardial contusion is likely in the context of blunt chest trauma.

Damage to the pericardium and myocardium is commonly seen after non-penetrating cardiac injuries. Traumatic pericarditis is characterized by the development of a friction rub and ST-T changes, whereas myocardial contusion confined to a small area of the myocardium often produces no significant symptoms or clinical signs. ST-T changes may be seen on the ECG.

Question 3.7: Answer

A Global concave ST elevation consistent with acute pericarditis and voltage criteria for left ventricular hypertrophy. There is a bifid P wave in II, evidence of left atrial enlargement.

Question 3.8: Answer

A Sinus rhythm with prolonged QT interval (550 ms). There is anterior T-wave inversion, possibly indicative of previous infarction. The P-wave morphology is consistent with right atrial enlargement. Note also the prominent R wave in V1. A positive QRS complex in V1 is associated with right ventricular hypertrophy, posterior infarction, WPW type A, RBBB, Duchenne's muscular dystrophy and incorrect precordial lead placement. In this patient old posterior infarction and right ventricular hypertrophy in the context of pulmonary hypertension are likely.

Question 3.9: Answer

A Acute inferior myocardial infarction with third-degree heart block and a ventricular escape rhythm of 48 bpm.

Complete heart block in the setting of an acute inferior wall infarction usually develops gradually, often progressing from first- to second-degree AV block. This form of AV block is usually transient and in the majority of patients resolves within a few days. In contrast, AV block in patients with an anterior wall infarction occurs rapidly and carries a high mortality.

Question 3.10: Answer

A

- Sinus rhythm with evidence of ventricular premature beats
- Biphasic P wave in V1 and peaked P wave in II suggestive of left and right atrial dilatation
- Left axis deviation and left anterior hemiblock
- Left ventricular hypertrophy.

Question 3.11: Answer

Sinus rhythm with first-degree heart block and profound bradycardia (HR ~38 bpm). Acute inferoseptal myocardial infarction.

Question 3.12: Answers

A There is diastolic equalization of central venous, pulmonary artery and wedge pressures consistent with pericardial tamponade, which may partly account for the observed low cardiac output.

B The CVP trace may reveal an absent 'y' descent. An echocardiograph would have revealed a pericardial effusion requiring drainage.

C Further fluid loading in the interim may be necessary to support the circulation. Attempts at reducing SVR may precipitate worsening hypotension in the presence of tamponade. His fever may represent sepsis, especially in the presence of invasive lines, but inadequate heat loss may also be a contributor. Pericardial effusion or haemorrhage should be considered in patients sustaining large infarcts who are subsequently given lysis or anticoagulated.

The development of cardiac tamponade in the setting of an acute MI may be related to pericardial haemorrhage secondary to pericarditis or to myocardial rupture within the first 3 days after an infarction. Both these conditions may be associated with cardiovascular collapse and shock. The presence of a large pericardial effusion in someone on anticoagulation after an acute infarct is an indication to discontinue anticoagulant therapy. Electromechanical dissociation and death usually follow tamponade secondary to ventricular rupture. Another condition which can present with hypotension, pulsus paradoxus and a raised JVP is massive right ventricular infarction. This can, however, be differentiated on echocardiography.

Question 3.13: Answer

A There is evidence of LV outflow tract obstruction related to hypertensive heart disease and left ventricular hypertrophy from aortic stenosis. Replacement of the aortic valve, functionally reducing the afterload, has resulted in systolic collapse of the subvalvular outflow tract and a significant pressure gradient. The principles of treatment consist of adequate fluid loading to maintain preload, ventricular relaxation with β-adrenergic antagonists or calcium channel antagonists, sequential AV pacing, and in severe cases maintenance of afterload with vasopressors. Occasionally a myomectomy or resection of the outflow tract may be warranted.

Question 3.14: Answer

A

- Heparin-induced thrombocytopoenia syndrome (HITS)

- Sepsis and hypersplenism causing reduced platelet lifespan

- Platelet destruction and haemolysis related to the prosthetic mitral valve, with the possibility of a paravalvular leak

- Other drugs, e.g. antibiotics (TMP-SMX), frusemide, thiazides, H_2-antagonists.

The presence of platelet Factor IV antibodies is strongly suggestive of HITS in a patient who has likely been exposed to prolonged heparin therapy related to cardiac surgery, valve anticoagulation and invasive haemodynamic monitoring. HITS is common in 1–3% of patients who receive unfractionated heparin for 7–14 days. The thrombocytopenia almost always begins 5–10 days after stopping heparin. The C14–serotonin release assay has been shown to have a high sensitivity and specificity for HIT antibodies.

In patients with suspected HITS, in whom anticoagulation is required, danaparoid sodium may be used.

Question 3.15: Answer

A The haemodynamic parameters suggest cardiogenic shock with associated low cardiac output, peripheral vasoconstriction, and what would normally be considered an adequate PAOP. There is also evidence of an elevated mixed venous SO_2 sampled from the pulmonary artery. This implies an intracardiac left -to-right shunt with a mixture of oxygenated and deoxygenated blood. In the context of an anteroseptal infarction this would be consistent with a ventricular septal defect (VSD), which could be confirmed by echocardiography.

Question 3.16: Answers

A There are ECG criteria supporting pulmonary hypertension: P pulmonale, right axis deviation and tall R waves in V1 with a right ventricular strain pattern. Cardiac catheter data show severely elevated pulmonary pressures consistent with chronic pulmonary hypertension. The transpulmonary pressure gradient is 54 mmHg and cardiac output is low, with a low PAOP, consistent with elevated pulmonary vascular resistance and satisfactory left ventricular function as the aetiology of this patient's symptoms. There is no evidence of a left-to-right shunt given a $PASO_2$ of 61%.

B There is reversibility demonstrated by a fall in PA pressures with 100% oxygen administration and a further significant decrease in pressures with inspired nitric oxide up to 38 ppm. The relevance is the possible clinical benefit to be expected from the commencement of calcium channel antagonists.

Question 3.17: Answers

A There is evidence of a left-to-right shunt, given the higher cardiac output measured with thermodilution than with the oesophageal doppler.

B The likely cardiac lesion is an atrial septal defect (ASD) because of equalization of atrial pressures.

C Other abnormalities include pulmonary hypertension and hyperdynamic circulation. There is also a significant response to nitric oxide with a reduction in PVRI and mean pulmonary artery pressures. PAM (mean pulmonary artery pressure) implies a component of potentially reversible vasoconstriction contributing to the high resistance . The high cardiac output is multifactorial: secondary to inotropes, probable L to R shunt increasing measured right heart cardiac output and hyperdynamic circulation due to sepsis.

Further reading

Datascope Clinical Support Services Department. Mechanics of Intra-Aortic Balloon Counterpulsation. Fairfield: Datascope Corp. 1997; USA

Gomez CMH, Palazzo MGA Pulmonary artery catheterization in anaesthesia and intensive care. Br J Anaesth. 1998; 81: 945–956

McLean AS Echocardiography Assessment of Left Ventricular Function in the Critically Ill. Anaesthesia and Intensive Care. 1996; 24(1): 60–65

Wagner GS Marriott's practical electrocardiography. 9th edn. Maryland: Williams & Wilkins, 1994; USA

Wojner AW Assessing the Five Points of the Intra-aortic Balloon Pump Waveform. Critical Care Nurse. 1994; 48–52

4

Respiratory mechanics, ventilation and oxygenation

Question 4.1

A 32-year-old woman sustained a closed fracture of the right distal radius and ulna yesterday. She had these reduced under intravenous regional analgesia with prilocaine 20 minutes ago. You are asked to review her with a view to admission to intensive care because she has become centrally and peripherally cyanosed following the procedure, and feels mildly breathless. On high-flow oxygen the pulse oximeter reads 88%. The arterial blood gases are as follows:

pH	7.46
PCO_2	32 mmHg
PO_2	326 mmol/L
HCO_3^-	22 mmHg

A What is the likely diagnosis?

B How can a definitive diagnosis be made?

C How will you manage this patient?

D What past medical history would significantly alter your management?

Question 4.2

A 40-year-old man, with a history of hepatitis C, presents with dyspnoea. On examination he is jaundiced, with spider naevi and ascites. Chest X-ray and spirometry are normal. Pulse oximetry (SpO_2) is performed:

Standing	88%
Supine	97%

A What is the likely diagnosis?

B What is the postulated pathophysiological mechanism?

C What further investigation is indicated?

D Is liver transplantation likely to help?

Question 4.3

A 46-year-old man presented with faecal peritonitis 2 weeks ago. He is now receiving TPN because of a generalized ileus. There is mild generalized weakness. He is afebrile. Current ventilator settings are CPAP 5 cmH$_2$O, pressure support 12 cmH$_2$O, FiO$_2$ 0.25.

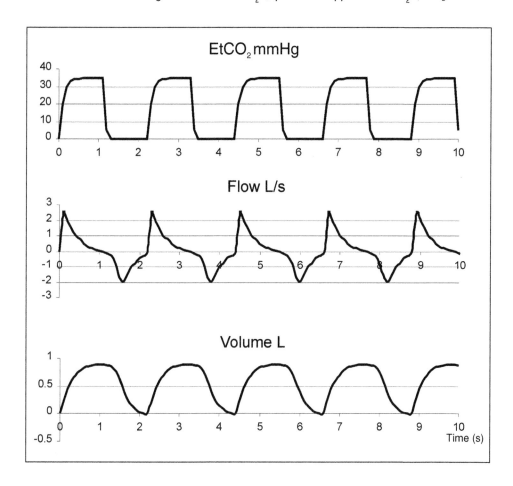

Arterial blood gases	
pH	7.42
EtCO$_2$	38 mmHg
PO$_2$	92 mmHg
HCO$_3^-$	24 mmol/L

A Suggest why this man is difficult to wean.

Question 4.4

A 36-year-old woman presents with 48 hours of cough and increasing shortness of breath. Chest X-ray shows alveolar infiltrates.

RFTs:	Actual	Predicted	95% CI
Spirometry			
FVC	2.23	3.64	(2.65–4.64)
FEV_1	1.97	2.86	(2.03–3.70)
FEV_1/FVC	88%	78%	
Diffusing capacity for carbon monoxide (DL_{CO})			
DL_{CO}	25.1	21.0	(15.0–27.0)
DL_{CO}/V_A	7.1	4.48	(2.63–6.32)

A Why do you think she is short of breath?

Question 4.5

A 60-year-old man presents with 5 years of increasing shortness of breath.

RFTs:	Actual	Predicted	95% CI
Spirometry			
FVC	1.32	4.32	(2.96–5.68)
FEV$_1$	1.12	3.08	(2.08–4.08)
FEV$_1$/FVC	85%	71%	
Plethysmography			
VC	1.35	4.32	(2.96–5.68)
TLC	2.37	6.18	(5.18–7.18)
RV	1.02	2.23	(1.44–3.02)
FRC	1.51	3.39	(2.68–4.10)
Diffusing capacity			
DL$_{CO}$	5.33	22.9	(14.7–31.1)
DL$_{CO}$/V$_A$	1.82	3.88	(2.04–5.72)

A Describe the results of the respiratory function tests and suggest one possible underlying diagnosis.

Question 4.6

A 62-year-old woman presents with 4 years of increasing shortness of breath.

RFTs:	Actual	Predicted	95% CI
Spirometry			
FVC	1.60	2.79	(1.80–3.78)
FEV$_1$	0.90	2.04	(1.20–2.87)
FEV$_1$/FVC	56%	73%	
Plethysmography			
VC	1.75	2.79	(1.80–3.78)
TLC	6.32	4.48	(3.71–5.24)
RV	4.57	1.70	(0.99–2.40)
FRC	5.2	2.71	(1.76–3.65)
Diffusing capacity			
DL$_{CO}$	9.2	17.1	(11.1–23.1)
DL$_{CO}$/V$_A$	1.1	3.83	(2.00–5.68)

A Describe the results of the respiratory function tests and suggest one possible underlying diagnosis.

Question 4.7

A 32-year-old man with shortness of breath on exercise for 2 years.

RFTs:	Actual	Predicted	95% CI
Spirometry			
FVC	3.21	5.32	(3.96–6.68)
FEV_1	2.76	1.00	(3.16–5.16)
FEV_1/FVC	86%	77.5%	
Plethysmography			
VC	3.37	5.32	(3.96–6.68)
TLC	6.52	7.08	(6.08–8.08)
RV	3.15	1.90	(1.11–2.69)
FRC	4.35	3.65	(2.94–4.36)
Helium dilution			
VC	3.41	5.32	(3.96–6.68)
TLC	5.04	7.08	(6.08–8.08)
RV	1.63	1.90	(1.11–2.69)
FRC	2.99	3.65	(2.94–4.36)

A What is the likely cause of the abnormalities on these respiratory function tests?

Question 4.8

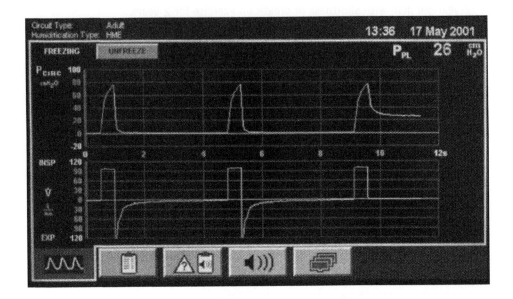

A 45-year-old woman presents with acute respiratory distress. On presentation she was obtunded. She was intubated and ventilated as an emergency. Shortly after intubation the ventilator shows these pressure and flow waveforms. Current ventilator settings: V_T 500 mL, rate 13 breaths/min, FiO_2 0.4, peak inspiratory flow rate 100 L/min.

A Suggest the likely cause of her respiratory failure. Give reasons.

Question 4.9

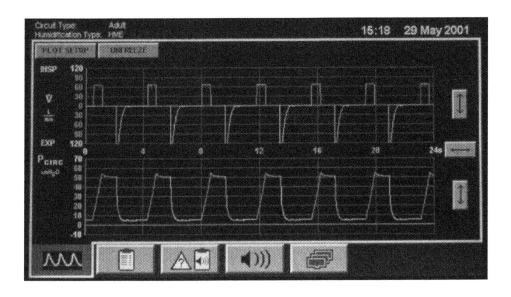

A 36-year-old woman was pulled unconscious from a swimming pool. She weighs 50 kg. She was intubated and ventilated. Shortly after intubation the ventilator shows these pressure and flow waveforms. Current ventilator settings: V_T 500 mL, rate 15 breaths/min, FiO_2 0.8, peak inspiratory flow rate 60 L/min. PaO_2 55 mmHg.

A What pulmonary pathology is likely to be present?

B What modifications will you make to the ventilator settings?

Question 4.10

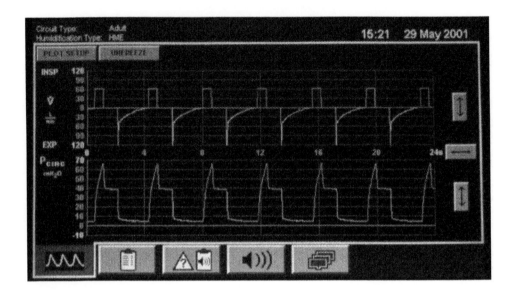

A 45-year-old man presents with increasing shortness of breath, hypoxaemic respiratory failure, and infiltrates on the chest X-ray. He weighs 80 kg. Current ventilator settings: V_T 500 mL, rate 15 breaths/min, FiO_2 0.5, peak inspiratory flow rate 60 L/min.

PaO_2 85 mmHg.

A Comment on the pressure and flow waveforms.

Question 4.11

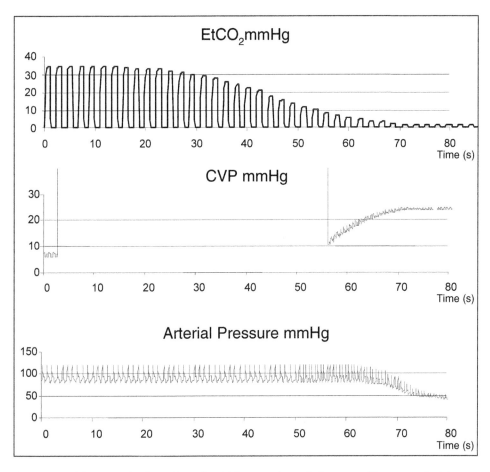

A 33-year-old woman had a subarachnoid haemorrhage 2 days ago. You are called to see her urgently because of the sudden profound hypotension.

A What is the most likely cause of the hypotension?

B What management will you undertake?

Question 4.12

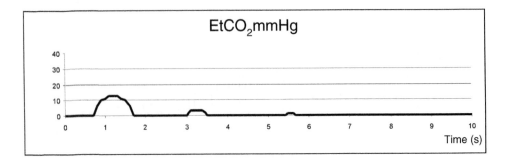

A 16-year-old woman is admitted with diazepam and paracetamol overdose. She requires airway protection because of depressed conscious level. She is intubated uneventfully, with a grade 1 laryngoscopy. Pulse oximetry shows SpO_2 = 100%, with a good waveform.

A Comment on the CO_2 waveform.

Question 4.13

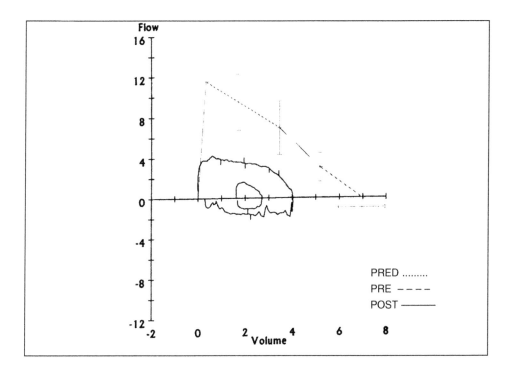

A 25-year-old man presents with 3 months of increasing shortness of breath on effort. Chest X-ray is clear. Height 195 cm, weight 100 kg.

RFTs:	Actual	Predicted	95% CI
Spirometry			
FVC	4.04	6.95	(5.94–7.96)
FEV$_1$	3.47	5.68	(4.72–6.64)
FEV$_1$/FVC	86%	82%	
PEF	4.21	11.51	
FEF$_{50\%}$	2.67	6.88	(9.95–4.21)
FIF$_{50\%}$	1.58		
FEF/FIF$_{50}$	2.17	<1.00	

A Describe the pattern of respiratory function tests and suggest one possible underlying diagnosis.

Question 4.14

A 36-year-old man has gas gangrene following an open ankle fracture. While in ICU he is ventilated with:

- 50% O_2, SIMV, PEEP 5 cmH$_2$O, V$_T$ 500 mL, rate 16

- Peak pressure 38 cmH$_2$O

- pH 7.33, PCO$_2$ 45 mmHg, HCO$_3$ 23 mmol/L, PO$_2$ 76 mmHg, SpO$_2$ 91%.

It is elected to treat him with hyperbaric oxygen. He is transported to the chamber and taken down to 2.8 atmospheres absolute. He rapidly becomes difficult to ventilate.

- 100% O_2, SIMV, PEEP 5, V$_T$ 500 mL, rate 16

- SpO$_2$ 71%, peak ventilatory pressure 60 cmH$_2$O (and failing to deliver set V$_T$)

- pH 7.12, PCO$_2$ 92 mmHg, HCO$_3$ 29 mmol/L, PO$_2$ 40 mmHg

A What are the likely causes for his deterioration?

B How will you manage this problem?

Question 4.15

A 27-year-old man with abdominal and chest trauma 2 days ago who currently has a right-sided haemopneumothorax, with moderate ongoing pleural air leak. Liver laceration being managed conservatively. SIMV FiO$_2$ 0.5, PEEP 5 cmH$_2$O, V$_T$ 800 ml, rate 16 bpm. Usually healthy and nutritional state is normal. Currently on nasogastric feeding 3000 mL/day of enteral nutrition with 1 kCal/mL.

Indirect calorimetry is performed to assess nutritional needs:

VO$_2$ 420, VCO$_2$ 336, RQ 0.8, total energy expenditure (TEE) 2000 kCal.

A Should the nutritional intake be altered based on this information?

Question 4.1: Answers

A Methaemoglobinaemia from prilocaine. Of all the local anaesthetic agents, prilocaine has by far the greatest propensity to cause methaemoglobinaemia.

B Multiple wavelength CO-oximetry demonstrates a high methaemoglobin fraction. High levels of methaemoglobinaemia tend to bias the pulse oximetry reading towards 85–90% value.

C Administration of oxygen, to ensure that the available haemoglobin is well saturated. If the patient has significant symptoms, then methylene blue may be administered as 1–2 mg/kg IV. If methylene blue is contraindicated or ineffective, exchange transfusion may be lifesaving. Hyperbaric oxygen, or ascorbic acid are other options.

D If there is a history of glucose-6-phosphate dehydrogenase deficiency, methylene blue should not be administered.

Question 4.2: Answers

A Hepatopulmonary syndrome in end-stage hepatitis C cirrhosis.

B Liver disease causes intrapulmonary vasodilation with R to L shunting. The process affects mainly the bases. Changes in posture that increase basal pulmonary blood flow (erect position) worsen gas exchange.

C Contrast echocardiography, injecting agitated saline intravenously. Delayed visualization of microbubbles in the left heart suggests intrapulmonary shunt, whereas immediate visualization would suggest intracardiac shunting.

D Yes. Over 80% of patients with hepatopulmonary syndrome have resolution or marked improvement in intrapulmonary vasodilatation with liver transplantation. This contrasts with portopulmonary hypertension, which is considered a contraindication.

Orthodeoxia is hypoxaemia accentuated in the erect position. Platypnoea is increased dyspnea in the erect position, improved by assuming the recumbent position. Causes include:

- Intracardiac shunts (intra-atrial shunt), with or without lung disease
- Pulmonary vascular shunts (pulmonary artery–pulmonary vein communications), either anatomical or parenchymal.

Question 4.3: Answer

A The ETCO$_2$ trace is normal apart from tachypnoea, and the a-ET CO$_2$ gradient is minimal, so significant rebreathing, $\dot{V}/\dot{Q}$ mismatch or dead space are unlikely. Given this, as the P_aCO_2 is normal and the minute (and hence the alveolar) ventilation is very high, CO$_2$ production must be high. In this clinical scenario the likely cause is overfeeding, in a patient with mild weakness who cannot cope with the minute ventilation demands required to maintain normocapnia without respiratory support.

Question 4.4: Answers

A Pulmonary haemorrhage. There is a mild restrictive defect and the DL$_{CO}$ is elevated from predicted, but within the normal range. However, when corrected for alveolar volume DL$_{CO}$ is significantly elevated.

B DL$_{CO}$ has two components, the membrane 'barrier to diffusion' and the rate of chemical combination of CO with haemoglobin in the pulmonary blood volume.

$$\frac{1}{DL_{CO}} = \frac{1}{DM_{CO}} + \frac{1}{Vc \times \theta_{CO}}$$

where DM$_{CO}$ is the diffusing capacity for CO through the alveolar capillary membrane, Vc is the pulmonary capillary blood volume, and θ_{CO} is the reaction rate of CO with haemoglobin. Blood in the alveolus takes up CO in the same way as blood in the pulmonary capillary, so DL$_{CO}$ rises as if pulmonary capillary blood volume were increased.

Question 4.5: Answer

A Restrictive pattern. There are many possible diagnoses, for example interstitial lung disease from asbestosis or idiopathic pulmonary fibrosis.

Question 4.6: Answer

A Obstructive pattern and reduced DL_{CO} suggests emphysema.

Question 4.7: Answer

A There is a restrictive picture on spirometry. RV and FRC measured by plethysmography are much higher than on He dilution, indicating significant gas trapping. As the spirometry is not an obstructive pattern, this suggests a pneumothorax or a bullous lung cyst. The 2-year history argues against a pneumothorax, so a lung cyst is the probable diagnosis.

Question 4.8: Answer

A Despite a relatively low tidal volume, the peak circuit pressures are very high. The plateau pressures (P_{pl}) are only minimally elevated. Expiration is prolonged, with the flow waveform not returning completely to baseline until after 3–4 seconds of expiration. This combination suggests severe airway obstruction. The level of dynamic hyperinflation is not severe because the P_{pl} is not markedly elevated, and the flow waveform returns to baseline. This woman has acute severe asthma.

The hyperinflation from incomplete exhalation leads to gas trapping and may be assessed during a period of apnoea long enough to allow complete exhalation of trapped gas. The pressure exerted on the alveolus from this trapped gas is termed auto-PEEP or intrinsic PEEP (PEEPi). The degree of hyperinflation can be estimated by:

- Plateau pressure (ideally maintained <20 cmH$_2$O)
- PEEPi maintained below 12 cmH$_2$O
- V_{EI} (end-inspiratory lung volume, which is the total exhaled volume during a period of apnoea, should be maintained <20 ml/kg).

Question 4.9: Answers

A The combination of high plateau pressures with minimal peak-plateau pressure gradient is indicative of poor lung compliance, and in this clinical setting ARDS from water inhalation is the most likely diagnosis.

B The plateau pressures are excessively high, putting her at risk of ventilator-induced lung injury (VALI). A tidal volume of 10 mL/kg is excessive in a patient with ARDS. The tidal volume should be reduced so the plateau pressure is <30–35 cmH_2O, and/or the VT reduced to 6 mL/kg to ameliorate VALI. This could be done with pressure control or volume control ventilation. PEEP should be increased to improve oxygenation, which may also minimize VALI though this is not proven.

Question 4.10: Answer

A There is a combined restrictive and obstructive pattern. The airway obstruction is suggested by the large difference between P_{peak} and P_{plat}. Compliance is 14.3 mL/cmH_2O, suggesting restrictive disease (see calculation of compliance below). The low compliance is not just due to overdistension from dynamic hyperinflation, because the expiratory flow waveform returns to zero before the onset of the following breath. This was a patient with extrinsic allergic alveolitis.

$$\text{Compliance} = \text{Tidal volume/inflation pressure}$$
$$= \text{Tidal volume/(plateau– extrinsic PEEP)}$$
$$= 500/(40\text{–}5) = 14.3 \text{ mL/cmH}_2\text{O}$$

Question 4.11: Answers

A Air embolus is suggested by a sudden deterioration during CVC manipulation, a fall in $EtCO_2$ before the hypotension and tachycardia. Patients with subarachnoid haemorrhage are commonly managed in a head-up position, particularly if intracranial hypertension is present. Another potential cause in this setting would be an anaphylactoid reaction.

B

- Head-down positioning
- Vasopressor/fluids/CPR if needed
- Consideration could be given to aspirating the CVC, which may remove some of the air load. Once the patient is resuscitated, consideration should be given to hyperbaric oxygen therapy.

Question 4.12: Answer

A The endotracheal tube is not in the trachea. With oesophageal intubation it is common for CO_2 to be measured during exhalation for a few breaths, particularly if the patient is hand ventilated prior to intubation.

Early detection of oesophageal intubation is the main reason that capnography should be used immediately following every intubation in the intensive care unit.

Question 4.13: Answer

A The flow/volume loop suggests a fixed large airway obstruction. Both inspiration and expiration are affected, with a flattening of the inspiratory and expiratory flow waveforms. The FEF/FIF_{50} is >1, demonstrating that inspiratory flow is affected more than expiratory. This suggests an extrathoracic site of obstruction. This man had an enlarged thyroid.

Question 4.14: Answers

A

• Pneumothorax needs to be considered, although it is a greater problem during decompression. If a trial of recompression improves the respiratory status, the clinical diagnosis is highly likely.

• Kinked or misplaced endotracheal tube is common during transport.

• Inadequate patient sedation and poor coordination with transport ventilator.

• Increased density of air under hyperbaric conditions may result in failure of delivery of tidal volume with some ventilators. Other ventilator malfunctions need to be considered.

B

• Hand ventilate with 100% O_2

• Sedate if appropriate

• Replace ETT if there is any doubt about its patency and correct placement

• Consider draining the chest if the above steps do not improve the problem. Chest X-ray is unlikely to be practical

• Do not surface until the problem is sorted out. He currently has PiO_2 of >1500 mmHg with critical oxygenation. Ascent will reduce FiO_2 and worsen any undrained pneumothorax.

Question 4.15: Answer

A Unless the patient is nutritionally depleted or obese, when nutrition is titrated against the results of indirect calorimetry the goal is to match caloric intake to total energy expenditure.

Indirect calorimetry is very sensitive to errors in measurement of gas volume and concentration. The technique is usually limited to FiO_2 of 0.6 or below, because of the inaccuracy of most sensors at high FiO_2. Leaks must be eliminated from the circuit.

There is a moderate ongoing pleural air leak, so the measured TEE of 2000 kCal is likely to be significantly less than the true TEE. Altering nutritional intake based on this information is not justified.

Further reading

Bilgin H, Ozcan B, Bilgin T Methemoglobinemia induced by methylene blue pertubation during laparoscopy. Acta Anaesthesiol Scand 1998; 42:594–595

Fallon MB, Abrams GA Pulmonary dysfunction in chronic liver disease. Hepatology 2000; 32:859–865

Golden PJ, Weinstein R Treatment of high-risk, refractory acquired methemoglobinemia with automated red blood cell exchange. J Clin Apheresis 1998; 13:28–31

Network TARDS Ventilation with lower tidal volumes as compared with traditional tidal volumes for acute lung injury and the acute respiratory distress syndrome. N Engl J Med 2000; 342:1301–1308

Nunn J Diffusion and alveolar capillary permeability. In: Nunn J, ed. Applied respiratory physiology. Oxford: Butterworth–Heinemann, 1993; 198–218

Nunn J Elastic forces and lung volumes. In: Nunn J, ed. Applied respiratory physiology. Oxford: Butterworth–Heinemann, 1993; 36–60

Reynolds KJ, Palayiwa E, Moyle JT, Sykes MK, Hahn CE The effect of dyshemoglobins on pulse oximetry: Part I, Theoretical approach and Part II, Experimental results using an in vitro test system. J Clin Monit 1993; 9:81–90

Robin ED, McCauley RF An analysis of platypnea–orthodeoxia syndrome including a "new" therapeutic approach. Chest 1997; 112:1449–1451

Smyrnios N, Curley F Indirect calorimetry. In: Rippe J, Irwin R, Fink M, Cerra F, eds. Intensive care medicine, 4th edn. Boston: Little, Brown & Co., 1996; 295–299

Tuxen D, Oh T Acute severe asthma. In: Oh T, ed. Intensive care manual, 4th edn. Oxford: Butterworth–Heinemann, 1997; 297–307

Wright RO, Lewander WJ, Woolf AD Methemoglobinemia: etiology, pharmacology, and clinical management. Ann Emerg Med 1999; 34:646–656

5.

Neurocritical care

Question 5.1

24 hours after head injury after a base of skull fracture. Bloodstained watery discharge from nose which tests positive for glucose.

A What is the likely diagnosis?

B How will you confirm the diagnosis?

Question 5.2

A 24-year-old Swedish woman working in Australia went on a weight loss programme. She was admitted to hospital with abdominal pain and distension. In the ward she became delirious, had a seizure and was found to become progressively weak, requiring intubation and ventilation.

O/E: HR 140/min, BP 170/110 Temp 38.5		
Abd: No bowel sounds		
CNS: No neck stiffness		
Motor power:		
Shoulders	3/5	
Hands	4/5	
Hips	3/5	
Ankles	5/5	
Reflexes	diminished	
Sensory	NAD	
Rest of clinical examination:	NAD	
Plasma sodium	124 mmol/L	(136–145)
LFT	Increased enzymes	
CSF	Normal	
FBC and blood picture	NAD	
Urine	Dark-coloured	

A What is the likely diagnosis?

B How will you confirm your diagnosis?

Question 5.3

A previously fit 35-year-old patient was admitted to the ICU with head and chest injuries following a motor vehicle accident (MVA). The patient had evidence of significant intracranial hypertension. In the first 48 hours after admission he was noted to have a large diuresis. The results of the blood and urine investigations are summarized below.

Sodium	142 mmol/L	(136–145)
Potassium	4.5 mmol/L	(3.5–5)
Urea	5.6 mmol/L	(3–8)
Creatinine	0.09 mmol/L	(0.04–0.12)
Glucose	6.8 mmol/L	(4–6)
Serum osmolality	327 mosm/kg	
Urine osmolality	324 mosm/kg	
Urine micro	1 WCC, no red cells	

A What is the likely explanation for the polyuria?

B Give reasons for your answer.

Question 5.4

A 28-year-old man with head injury – day 3.

ICP (intracranial pressure)	33 mmHg	
MAP (mean arterial pressure)	90 mmHg	
Jugular bulb saturation (SjO$_2$)	51%	(55–75%)
Arterial pH	7.55	(7.36–7.44)
PCO$_2$	27 mmHg	(36–44)
PO$_2$	94 mmHg	(90–110)
SaO$_2$	99%	

A List four abnormalities.

B List your responses in sequence to the SjO$_2$ measurement.

Question 5.5

A 36-year-old woman who has been in hospital for 10 days after an LSCS now develops weakness of the face, arms and legs. GCS 15. Pupils fixed and dilated. Tone: symmetrically reduced, reflexes diminished bilaterally. Sensory examination is normal.

FBC	NAD	
ELFT	NAD	
CT brain	NAD	
MRI brain	NAD	
CSF		
Cells	2/mm³	
Protein	200 mg/L	(150–400)
Glucose	2.2 mmol/L	

A What is your differential diagnosis?

Question 5.6

A 23-year-old woman was brought into casualty in an unconscious state. Pupils equal and reactive. No lateralizing signs on neurological examination.

CT brain scan:	NAD	
CSF studies:	NAD	
Venous blood		
Sodium	137 mmol/L	(137–145)
Potassium	3.1 mmol/L	(3.1–4.2)
Chloride	115 mmol/L	(101–109)
Bicarbonate	28 mmol/L	(22–32)
Urea	7.0 mmol/L	(3.0–8.0)
Creatinine	0.08 mmol/L	(0.05–0.12)
Total protein	80 g/L	(65–80)
Albumin	34 g/L	(39–50)
Calcium	2.3 mmol/L	(2.2–2.65)

A Suggest a likely diagnosis; give one reason.

Question 5.1: Answers

A Cerebrospinal fluid rhinorrhoea

B Test for β_2-transferrin. Traditionally, the detection of glucose in the clear fluid draining from the nose, ear or orbit was considered diagnostic of a CSF leak. This test has a number of false positives and has now been replaced by the β_2-transferrin assay (previously known as the τ protein), which is highly specific for CSF. Transferrin is an iron-binding glycoprotein synthesized primarily in the liver. In the CSF, two isoforms are found, β_1-transferrin (same as serum) and β_2-transferrin. The latter is absent in the serum and is formed in the CSF from its β_1 analogue by the action of CSF neuraminidase. It is therefore specific for the CSF and its presence has been used as a diagnostic test to detect CSF leakage.

Question 5.2: Answers

A Acute intermittent porphyria. The differential diagnosis of a rapid-onset motor neuropathy includes Guillain–Barré syndrome, transverse myelitis, poliomyelitis, snake bite, botulism and porphyria. The presence of abdominal pain, seizures and a normal CSF examination exclude the first three possibilities. The features in the history are also inconsistent with snake bite. Botulism presents with a typical descending paralysis and autonomic involvement. The presence of hyponatraemia, dark-coloured urine and a rapid-onset motor neuropathy suggests the diagnosis of acute intermittent porphyria. Starvation and anticonvulsants are well known triggers. The mechanism of hyponatraemia is unclear. Increased ADH levels, GI loss of sodium and a sodium-losing nephropathy have been described.

B Urine for porphyrins

Question 5.3: Answers

A Mannitol administration

B The differential diagnoses of polyuria in the acute phase of head injury include cranial diabetes insipidus (DI), alcohol intoxication prior to the accident, cerebral salt-wasting syndrome (CSW) and mannitol administration. DI is characterized by a high serum osmolality, low urine osmolality and a hypernatraemia. In this patient the urine osmolality was in the normal range. Closer inspection of the data reveals an osmolar gap of 30. The osmolar gap is the difference between the measured and calculated osmolality. A value >20 represents an elevated osmolar gap and suggests the presence of osmotically active solutes such as the alcohols or mannitol. CSW is not associated with an elevated osmolar gap. Alcohol is unlikely to be present in the circulation 48 hours after admission to the intensive care unit. The most likely explanation for the polyuria is mannitol administration.

Question 5.4: Answers

A High ICP, low CPP (57 mmHg), jugular bulb desaturation, hypocapnia, respiratory alkalosis

B Check accuracy of reading by drawing a sample of blood from the jugular bulb and measuring its oxygen saturation in a CO-oximeter. If it is a true desaturation, this implies either a reduction in oxygen delivery to the brain or an increase in oxygen consumption by the brain. To improve oxygen delivery, the measures to be taken include:

- Decrease ventilatory rate to maintain $PaCO_2$ between 35 and 40 mmHg to avoid hypocapnia-induced cerebral vasoconstriction

- Control ICP to improve CPP

- Increase fluids/inotropes to augment MAP and CPP.

To reduce oxygen consumption by the brain:

- Control temperature

- Control seizure activity, if any.

Jugular bulb saturation: Interpretation

55–75%	Normal range
50–55%	Critical SjO_2
<50%	Pathological
>75%	Hyperaemia

Approach to jugular bulb desaturation (SjO_2 <50%)

(a) Check accuracy of reading by CO-oximetry

(b) Check ABG, correct low PO_2

(c) Check MAP; if low, correct

(d) Check Hb; if low, treat

(e) Check ICP; if high, treat

(f) Check electrical activity to exclude fitting

Approach to jugular bulb hyperaemia (SjO_2 >75%)

(a) Check accuracy of reading by CO-oximetry

(b) If increased CBF is contributory – check PCO_2

(c) If decreased cerebral oxygen consumption is contributory check ICP, consider CT

Question 5.5: Answer

A The differential diagnosis of this presentation would include some of the causes of a pure motor neuropathy. These include postoperative Guillain–Barré syndrome, myasthenia gravis, porphyria and wound botulism. Snake bite, tick paralysis, toxins and infestations are unlikely 10 days into hospitalization. Guillain–Barré syndrome is unlikely in the setting of fixed dilated pupils and a normal CSF protein, though pupillary abnormalities can occur, and the CSF protein can be normal in the initial stages. Myasthenia gravis would not normally cause fixed dilated pupils and the hyporeflexia argues against it. In the absence of any seizures, mental changes, electrolyte abnormalities and discoloration of urine, porphyria is unlikely. Rarely an acute stroke could present with flaccid weakness of the arms and legs; however with normal mentation and imaging, that is unlikely. Wound botulism has been described, classically in the postoperative setting, and appears to present 10 days after surgery. The features include lower motor neuron type weakness, normal sensation and pupillary involvement. Bulbar palsy is almost always present, with the four Ds: dysphonia, dysphagia, diplopia, dysarthria. There are three characteristic features: symmetric, descending flaccid paralysis with prominent bulbar palsies; in an afebrile patient; with a clear sensorium.

Question 5.6: Answer

A Lithium overdose. The calculated anion gap is in fact –6. A low or a negative anion gap would suggest the presence of hypoalbuminaemia (albumin levels are normal in this patient), hypercalcaemia, hypermagnesaemia, hyperglobulinaemia and lithium intoxication. Hypermagnesaemia is unlikely in someone with normal renal function.

Further reading

De Deyne C, Van Aken J, Decruyenaere J, Struys M, Colardyn F Jugular bulb oximetry: review on a cerebral monitoring technique. Acta Anaesthesiol Belg 1998; 49:21–31

Ryall RG, Peacock MK, Simpson DA Usefulness of beta 2-transferrin assay in the detection of cerebrospinal fluid leaks following head injury. J Neurosurg 1992; 77:737–739

Timmer RT, Sands JM. Lithium intoxication. J Am Soc Nephrol 1999; 10:666–674

Venkatesh B, Scott P, Ziegenfuss M Cerebrospinal fluid in critical illness. Crit Care Resusc 2000; 2:43–55

6

Microbiology

Question 6.1

A 31-year-old diabetic woman presents with headache and facial pain. She has become mildly confused over the last 6 hours and is febrile. There is a black necrotic lesion on the hard palate. There is proptosis of the left eye and black fluid is draining from the orbit.

Blood gases/blood glucose/urinary ketones:

Arterial blood gas ($FiO_2 = 0.21$)		
pH	7.22	(7.35–7.45)
PCO_2	20 mmHg	(35–45)
Bicarbonate	8 mEq/L	(22–33)
PO_2	109 mmHg	(80–100)
Glucose	24 mmol/L	(3–7.8)
Urine: Ketones +++		

A What is the likely cause of her illness?

B What is the most common causative microorganism?

C What management is indicated?

Question 6.2

A 45-year-old man has been holidaying in the Northern Territory of Australia during the wet season. In the last 24 hours he developed fever, cough and myalgia. He is mildly confused, and has marked muscle tenderness. Intubation and ventilation is required because of rapidly progressive hypoxaemic respiratory failure. Tracheal aspirate shows Gram-negative bacilli.

A What will you use for your initial antibiotic therapy, before culture results are available?

B What is the most likely causative organism?

Question 6.3

A 42-year-old man has had a cough for 2 weeks. He now presents with fever and a mild left hemiparesis. CT scan of the head demonstrates a lesion in the right frontal lobe. A stereotactic biopsy is undertaken.

Gram stain shows weakly Gram-positive beaded branching filaments which are weakly acid fast.

A What is the likely causative organism?

B What antibiotic therapy should be used?

Question 6.4

A 26-year-old man presents with shortness of breath, confusion, fever and hypotension. CXR shows lobar pneumonia. Sputum sample shows Gram-positive diplococci.

Venous blood

WBC	22 × 10⁹/L	(4.0–10.5)
Hgb	146 g/L	(130–170)
Platelets	978 × 10⁹/L	(150–400)
Neutrophils	17.8 × 10⁹/L	(1.9–6.8)
Lymphocytes	2.1 × 10⁹/L	(1.2–3.7)
Eosinophils	0.5 × 10⁹/L	(0.0–0.8)
Monocytes	1.2 × 10⁹/L	(0.2–0.8)

Moderate anisocytosis. Slight poikilocytosis. Occasional target cells. Occasional stomatocytes. Moderate number of Howell–Jolly bodies.

A What organism is likely to be causing this illness?

B Suggest why he is predisposed to this illness.

C What measure could have been undertaken to attempt to prevent this illness?

Question 6.5

A 55-year-old hepatitis C-positive woman with known chronic liver disease presents with neck stiffness and drowsiness.

CSF		
WBC	90×10^6/L (<5)	70% neutrophils
RBC	1×10^6/L (<5)	
Protein	0.6 mg/L	(0.15–0.4)
Glucose	1.1 mmol/L (2.8–4.0)	(plasma glucose 3.8)
Gram stain	No organisms seen	
Blood culture	Gram-positive bacilli	

A What is the likely diagnosis?

B What would be suitable antibiotic therapy for the likely organism?

Question 6.6

A 3-year-old child has had diarrhoea and fever for 1 week, which are now settling. Her mother brings her to hospital because she is lethargic and irritable.

Venous blood

Sodium	145 mmol/L	(135–145)
Potassium	5.6 mmol/L	(3.2–4.5)
Urea	35.2 mmol/L	(3.0–8.0)
Creatinine	0.32 mmol/L	(0.05–0.10)
Bilirubin	48 μmol/L	(3–17)
WBC	8.0 × 10^9/L	(5.5–15.5)
Hgb	88 g/L	(130–170)
Platelets	48 × 10^9/L	(150–400)
Neutophils	5.1 × 10^9/L	(1.5–8.5)
Lymphocytes	2.1 × 10^9/L	(2.0–8.0)
Eosinophils	0.5 × 10^9/L	(0.02–0.65)
Monocytes	0.5 × 10^9/L	(0.0–0.8)
Reticulocytes	3.0 × 10^9/L	(0.0–1.0)

Schistocytes, occasional spherocytes.

A What is the likely diagnosis?

B What is the likely cause of the diarrhoea?

Question 6.7

A 27-year-old woman returned home from a diving holiday in New Guinea 48 hours ago. Yesterday she became febrile with rigors; today she is comatosed and fitting.

Venous blood

Sodium	140 mmol/L	(135–145)
Potassium	4.9 mmol/L	(3.2–4.5)
Urea	40.2 mmol/L	(3.0–8.0)
Creatinine	0.41 mmol/L	(0.05–0.10)
Bilirubin	50 μmol/L	(3–17)
LDH	500 U/L	(110–250)
Glucose	2.4 mmol/L	(3.0–7.8)
WBC	15.0×10^9/L	(4.0–12.0)
Hgb	75 g/L	(120–160)
Platelets	35×10^9/L	(150–400)
Neutrophils	$5.1 \times x \times 10^9$/L	(1.5–8.5)
Lymphocytes	2.1×10^9/L	(2.0–8.0)
Eosinophils	0.5×10^9/L	(0.02–0.65)
Monocytes	0.5×10^9/L	(0.0–0.8)
Reticulocytes	3.0×10^9/L	(0.0–1.0)

A What is your working diagnosis?

B What investigation will you order to confirm the diagnosis?

C If your diagnosis is confirmed, what treatment will you initiate?

D Should steroids be given?

Question 6.8

A 48 year old man presented with severe flank pain, fevers and rigors. On presentation the pulse was 130/min and the blood pressure 60/20. Urinary microscopy showed >500 × 10^6/L leukocytes, with +++ bacteria. 10 L of normal saline and an adrenaline (epinephrine) infusion (30 µg/min) were administered, and BP rose to 100/60. He required intubation and ventilation for deteriorating gas exchange.

A What are the likely possibilities for a causative microorganism?

B What urgent radiological investigation is indicated?

C What would be the indications for urgent surgery or radiological intervention in this unstable patient?

Question 6.9

A 48-year-old man presents with 1 week of non-productive cough, fevers and increasing shortness of breath. Medications include diclofenac, methotrexate and prednisolone, which he has been taking in a dose of 25 mg/day for 12 months to treat severe rheumatoid arthritis affecting his knees and hands. Chest X-Ray shows bilateral diffuse interstitial infiltrates. SpO_2 73% on 6 L O_2 via a Hudson mask. Following intubation and ventilation a bronchoalveolar lavage (BAL) is performed. Gram stain and cultures are negative.

A What is the likely causative micro-organism?

B How will you confirm the diagnosis ?

C What antibiotic should be used, in what dose, and for how long?

D Suggest an alternative agent if side effects occur with the first agent.

E What coexisting infection should be looked for?

F What is the role for steroids in this condition?

Question 6.10

A 32-year-old woman presented with 48 hours of cough, fevers, rigors and increasing shortness of breath, with bronchial breathing at the right lung base. Chest X-ray showed dense consolidation of the right lower lobe. Blood and sputum cultures grew *Streptococcus pneumoniae*. Treatment with intravenous benzylpenicillin 1.2 g, 4 hourly, continues. She was intubated and ventilated on arrival in hospital 5 days ago, and is deteriorating. With FiO_2 0.9, pressure control ventilation, PIP 30 cmH$_2$O, PEEP 15 cmH$_2$O, I:E ratio 2:1, the PaO_2 is only 55 mmHg. Chest X-ray now shows bilateral alveolar infiltrates consistent with ARDS. She has high fevers and the WBC is 25 × 10^9/L.

A Suggest reasons why she may not be improving

Question 6.11

A 32-year-old woman presents with low-grade fever, headache and confusion.

CSF			
WBC	$50 \times 10^6/L$	(<5)	90% lymphocytes
RBC	$1 \times 10^6/L$	(<5)	
Protein	0.47 mg/L	(0.15–0.4)	
Glucose	4.2 mmol/L	(Plasma glucose 4.8)	
Gram stain	No organisms seen		

A What diagnoses need to be considered?

B What further investigations will you perform?

C What therapy will you start pending the results of further investigations?

Question 6.12

A 56-year-old man presents with pyelonephritis. Empirically treated with ceftriaxone 1 g daily. Ultrasound reveals an obstructed right kidney. Percutaneous nephrostomy is performed.

Blood cultures: 2/2 bottles growing *Enterobacter cloacae*, sensitive to ceftriaxone

Pus from renal pelvis: Gram-negative bacillus on microscopy. Cultures growing *Enterobacter cloacae*, sensitive to ceftriaxone

A Comment on the antibiotic therapy.

Question 6.13

A 28-year-old woman presents with a 3-day history of fever, cough, sore throat and earache. On chest auscultation there are bilateral crackles. There are skin lesions suggestive of erythema multiforme.

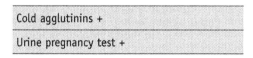

Cold agglutinins +
Urine pregnancy test +

A What is your working diagnosis?

B What therapy will you start?

Question 6.14

A 68-year-old man cut his foot on a shell while on holiday at a subtropical seaside resort. Over the next 48 hours mild cellulitis developed around the cuts, which have ulcerated. The following day this rapidly developed into a fulminant necrotizing cellulitis over most of his lower limbs. He is profoundly shocked.

Blood cultures at 24 hours: 2 out of 2 bottles growing Gram-negative bacilli

A What is the likely pathogen?

B What antibiotic therapy will you use pending sensitivity results?

Question 6.15

A 32-year-old male presents with 1 week of confusion and a seizure on the day of presentation. He is an intravenous drug user who has had fevers and lost weight over the last 3 months. Generalized lymphadenopathy is present. CT scan shows multiple bilateral cerebral lesions, with involvement of the basal ganglia. The lesions are hypodense, with ring enhancement after i.v. contrast.

A What is the most likely cause of the cerebral lesions?

B Suggest why the patient may be prone to this problem.

C What important differential diagnosis should be considered?

D What therapy will you initiate?

Question 6.1: Answers

A Rhinocerebral mucormycosis.

B Mucormycosis is caused by moulds of the order Mucorales. The most common species is *Rhizopus arrhizus*.

C Correction of diabetic ketoacidosis. Surgical debridement. Amphotericin B (preferably liposomal in high dose).

Question 6.2: Answers

A In addition to conventional treatment for community-acquired pneumonia cover (for example erythromycin and ceftriaxone), the therapy should be broadened to Should included cover for melioidosis (meropenem or ceftazidime plus co-trimoxazole).

B *Burkholderia pseudomallei* (previously *Pseudomonas pseudomallei*). Melioidosis is endemic in southeast Asia and northern Australia. Infections caused by *Burkholderia pseudomallei* constitute a broad spectrum of acute and chronic, local and systemic, clinical and subclinical disease processes collectively called *melioidosis*. Acute pulmonary disease may result in the septicaemic form of melioidosis, which may follow a rapid downhill course and result in death unless aggressive therapy is instituted.

Question 6.3: Answers

A *Nocardia* sp., most commonly *Nocardia asteroides*. Clinical manifestations of CNS nocardiosis result from granulomas or abscesses in the brain, and less commonly in the spinal cord or the meninges.

B Trimethoprim-sulphamethoxazole (co-trimoxazole) is usually recommended. It is the treatment of choice for infections caused by N. *brasiliensis and N. asteroides complex*. For those with sulphonamide intolerance or in those with N. *otitidiscavarium* infection, alternative regimens include amikacin, imipenem and third-generation cephalosporins.

Question 6.4: Answers

A *Streptococcus pneumoniae.* Pneumococcus is the organism most commonly (50–90%) implicated in postsplenectomy sepsis (PSS). Infections by *H. influenzae* type B, *N. meningitidis*, *Capnocytophaga canimorsus* and *Salmonella* also occur with increased frequency in asplenic patients.

B Previous splenectomy, as indicated by Howell–Jolly bodies on his blood picture and thrombocytosis. One to two percent of individuals, who have suffered post-traumatic asplenia develop an episode of PSS. The timing of PSS in relation splenectomy remains unclear. However in a retrospective review of PSS, 32% occurred in the first year after splenectomy and 52% within 2 years. The younger the patient at the time of splenectomy, the shorter the time interval to PSS. About a third of these patients have an episode of PSS within the first year, and 50% by the second year after splenectomy.

C Pneumococcal vaccination +/– penicillin. Pneumococcal immunization is recommended for the asplenic or the hyposplenic patient.

Whilst there are data to show that this vaccine confers protection in hyposplenic individuals, anecdotal reports of failures do exist.

Penicillin prophylaxis is commonly used in the hyposplenic paediatric population, particularly in those with sickle cell anaemia for a period of 2 years. Long-term penicillin prophylaxis in splenectomized adults is generally not recommended.

Question 6.5: Answers

A An immunocompromised patient with Gram-positive bacilli meningitis suggests *Listeria monocytogenes* as the causative organism. The term monocytogenes refers to the monocytosis that is frequently seen in rabbits with this condition, but which is uncommon in humans. The clinical features peculiar to *Listeria* meningitis include:

- Neck stiffness only present in 80% of patients

- A higher incidence of seizures and movement disorders

- Fluctuating sensorium

- Blood cultures are more frequently positive

- CSF findings: normal CSF glucose in >60% of patients and a frequently negative Gram stain.

B Ampicillin or penicillin are suitable agents. For those with penicillin allergy, trimethoprim-sulphamethoxazole may be used. Cephalosporins are not useful in the treatment of *Listeria* meningitis.

Question 6.6: Answers

A Haemolytic–uraemic syndrome.

B Enterohaemorrhagic *E. coli*; the most common type worldwide is O157:H7.

Question 6.7: Answers

A The most likely diagnosis is *Plasmodium falciparium* cerebral malaria, given the history and the severity of the clinical and laboratory findings.

B Microscopic examination of thick and thin blood smear. ELISA for parasite antigen or PCR also have similar (or greater) sensitivity.

C Intravenous quinine (or quinidine) is probably the best choice. An alternative is an artemisinin derivative (artemether or artsunate) followed by a supplementary drug to prevent recurrence. Chloroquine is not suitable, given the high chloroquine resistance in this area.

D No. Steroids worsen the outcome of cerebral malaria.

Question 6.8: Answers

A *Escherichia coli, Proteus, Pseudomonas, Klebsiella, Enterobacter, Enterococcus.*

B Urgent ultrasound or CT to exclude an obstructed urinary tract.

C

• Obstructed ureter with pyonephrosis (nephrostomy or ureteric stent)

• Emphysematous pyelonephritis (nephrectomy)

• Intrarenal or perinephric abscess (percutaneous drainage initially).

Question 6.9: Answers

A *Pneumocystis carinii* pneumonia.

B Giemsa and methenamine silver stains from the BAL fluid are positive. PCR for pneumocystis on the BAL fluid.

C Cotrimoxazole as trimethoprim (15–20 mg/kg/day) and sulphamethaxaxole (70–150 mg/kg/day) in 3–4 divided doses. A treatment course of 2 weeks is usual for non-HIV patients and 3 weeks in HIV patients, but long-term secondary prophylaxis is required for all patients who survive *Pneumocystis carinii* pneumonia.

D Pentamidine isethionate.

E HIV.

F Patients with moderate to severe pneumocystis in the context of HIV benefit from the early use of steroids. The role of steroids in non-HIV patients is not as well proven, but they are often used.

Question 6.10: Answer

A

- Resistant organism. Penicillin resistance is becoming increasingly common in pneumococci. Although precise data on the proportion of pneumococci exhibiting penicillin susceptibility are not available, studies from North America suggest that this figure ranges from 40 to 80%. Intermediate resistance is defined as MIC of 0.1–1 µg/mL, and these strains are readily treated with higher doses of penicillin. Alternative antibiotics should be used for highly resistant strains (MIC ≥ 2.0 µg/mL). Highly resistant strains of pneumococci still remain susceptible to vancomycin and/or fluoroquinolones.

- Underlying immunodeficiency. Pneumococcal infection is more common in patients with congenital or acquired agammaglobulinaemia, multiple myeloma, lymphoma, chronic lymphocytic leukaemia, HIV, hyposplenism and complement deficiencies.

- Nosocomial infection. Examples include line sepsis, urinary tract infection, sinusitis from nasogastric tube.

- Pneumococcal infection that is localized may not respond to antibiotic therapy alone, and surgery may be needed (empyema is the most common, followed by endocarditis, septic arthritis, sinusitis).

- A second pathology – left ventricular failure due to occult mitral stenosis – may be precipitated by the haemodynamic changes of sepsis.

Question 6.11: Answers

A

- Viral meningoencephalitis. *Herpes simplex* is the most likely, though other forms of flavivirus and HIV may cause this picture
- Partially treated bacterial meningitis
- Chronic meningoencephalitis such as TB, syphilis or cryptococcus
- Cerebral lymphoma.

B

- MRI, viral culture, herpes PCR on CSF
- Bacterial PCR on the CSF
- Cryptococcal antigen
- Depending on other clinical features consideration may be given to: Ziehl–Nelsen stain, TB culture, syphilis serology, cytology, and viral serology including HIV.

C 10 mg/kg i.v. aciclovir 8 hourly.

Question 6.12: Answer

A *Enterobacter cloacae* is a member of the ESCAPPM group of organisms, which include *Enterobacter, Serratia, Citrobacter freundii, Acinetobacter, Providencia, Pseudomonas* and *Morganella*.

These organisms have an inducible chromosomally encoded cephalosporinase (a Bush group 1 β-lactamase). Emergence of this form of resistance (to all currently available cephalosporins) is frequent when these organisms are treated with broad-spectrum cephalosporins, and often translates to clinical failure of the β-lactam therapy.

Question 6.13: Answers

A The clinical picture suggests *Mycoplasma pneumoniae* infection. Cold agglutinins occur in 50–70% of patients. A wide variety of skin conditions have been reported in *M. pneumoniae* infection. Erythema multiforme occurs in up to 7% of patients.

B Tetracycline or a macrolide are usually used as therapy. Tetracycline is contraindicated in this patient because of her pregnancy.

Question 6.14: Answer

A *Vibrio vulnificus* (and *V. alginolyticus*) should be considered. This organism has been implicated in otherwise healthy people, with the rapid development of intense cellulitis, necrotizing vasculitis and ulcer formation, and is often associated with bacteraemia after contamination of a superficial wound with warm seawater. Other risk factors for the development of this infection include the consumption of raw oysters, liver disease and iron overload states.

B In this clinical scenario broad-spectrum Gram-negative cover is appropriate, but *V. vulnificus* is not universally susceptible to aminoglycosides. Tetracyclines are first choice for therapy for *V. vulnificus* and should be included in the antibiotic regimen. Cefotaxime and ciprofloxacin are alternatives.

Question 6.15: Answers

A *Toxoplasma gondii* infection is the most likely cause of the cerebral lesions, given the clinical features suggestive of AIDS.

B There is a high probability that the patient has an underlying HIV infection.

C An important differential to consider is cerebral lymphoma, which may be confused with cerebral toxoplasmosis in the HIV patient.

D Recommended therapy is pyrimethamine (combined with folinic acid to reduce the incidence of pyrimethamine-associated myelotoxicity) and either sulfadiazine or clindamycin. If HIV infection is confirmed, antiretroviral therapy is also indicated.

Further reading

Baum S *Mycoplasma pneumoniae* and atypical pneumonia. In: Mandell G, Bennett J, Dolin R, eds. Principles and practice of infectious diseases. New York: Churchill Livingstone, 2000; 2018–2026

Corey L Herpes simplex virus. In: Mandell G, Bennett J, Dolin R, eds. Principles and practice of infectious diseases. New York: Churchill Livingstone, 2000; 1564–1580

Filice G Nocardiosis. In: Isselbacher K et al., eds. Principles of internal medicine, 13th edn. New York: McGraw Hill, 1994; 696–698

French M HIV infection and the acquired immunodeficiency syndrome. In: Oh T, ed. Intensive care manual, 4th ed. Oxford: Butterworth–Heinemann, 1997:522

Krogstad D *Plasmodium* species (Malaria). In: Mandell G, Bennett J, Dolin R, eds. Principles and practice of infectious diseases. New York: Churchill Livingstone, 2000; 2817–2831

Lutwick L Infections in asplenic patients. In: Mandell G, Bennett J, Dolin R, eds. Principles and practice of infectious diseases. New York: Churchill Livingstone, 2000; 3169–3176

McArthur C, Judson J Abdominal and pelvic injuries. In: Oh T, ed. Intensive care manual. 4th ed. Oxford: Butterworth–Heinemann, 1997:608

Musher D *Streptococcus pneumoniae*. In: Mandell G, Bennett J, Dolin R, eds. Principles and practice of infectious diseases. New York: Churchill Livingstone, 2000; 2128–2147

Neill M, Carpenter C Other pathogenic vibrios. In: Mandell G, Bennett J, Dolin R, eds. Principles and practice of infectious diseases. New York: Churchill Livingstone, 2000; 2274

Opal S, Mayer K, Medeiros A Mechanisms of bacterial antibiotic resistance. In: Mandell G, Bennett J, Dolin R, eds. Principles and practice of infectious diseases. New York: Churchill Livingstone, 2000; 236–252

Pollack M.*Pseudomonas* infections. In: Isselbacher K et al., eds. Principles of internal medicine, 13th edn. New York: McGraw Hill, 1994; 670–71

Rondeau E, Peraldi MN *Escherichia coli* and the hemolytic–uremic syndrome. N Engl J Med 1996; 335:660–662

Schuchat A, Broome C Infections caused by *Listeria Monocytogenes*. In: Isselbacher K et al., eds. Principles of internal medicine, 13th edn. New York: McGraw Hill, 1994; 631–632

Sobel J, Kaye D Urinary tract infections. In: Mandell G, Bennett J, Dolin R, eds. Principles and practice of infectious diseases. New York: Churchill Livingstone, 2000; 773–805

Sugar A Agents of mucormycosis and related species. In: Mandell G, Bennett J, Dolin R, eds. Principles and practice of infectious diseases. New York: Churchill Livingstone, 2000; 2685–2691

Walzer P *Pneumocystis carinii*. In: Mandell G, Bennett J, Dolin R, eds. Principles and practice of infectious diseases. New York: Churchill Livingstone, 2000; 2781–2795

7

Coagulation abnormalities

Question 7.1

60-year-old man with alcoholic cirrhosis is diagnosed with bacterial endocarditis.

INR	2.4	(0.9–1.3)
PT	27 s	(9–14)
APTT	21 s	(25–38)
TCT	12 s	(12–18)
Echis time	15 s	(11–18)

A What is the nature of the observed coagulopathy?

Question 7.2

An 85-year-old woman presents with a ruptured oesophagus and empyema. A jejunostomy feeding tube is in situ.

INR	2.0	(0.9–1.3)
PT	21 s	(9–14)
APTT	35 s	(25–38)
TCT	18 s	(12–18)
Echis time	20 s	(11–18)
Fibrinogen	1.4 g/L	(1.5–4.0)
Platelets	160 x 10⁹/L	(140–400)

A What is the nature of her coagulopathy?

Question 7.3

A 54-year-old man returns from theatre post CABG (coronary artery bypass grafting) and is bleeding briskly into the chest drains.

INR	1.4	(0.9–1.3)
PT	16 s	(9–14)
APTT	55 s	(25–38)
TCT	17 s	(12–18)
Fibrinogen	1.2 g/L	(1.5–4.0)
Platelets	65 x 10⁹/L	(140–400)

A How would you correct this man's coagulation profile?

Question 7.4

A 55-year-old woman presents for a lobectomy because of carcinoma. Her preoperative coagulation screen is as follows:

INR	1.2	(0.9–1.3)
PT	15 s	(9–14)
APTT	49 s	(25–38)
APTT 50% NP	46 s	(25–38)
TCT	16 s	(12–18)
Fibrinogen	3.1 g/L	(1.5–4.0)
Platelets	127 x 10⁹/L	(140–400)

(APTT 50% NP implies APTT values after mixing patient's sample with pooled normal plasma – 50:50 mix.)

A Interpret the coagulation profile and suggest possible diagnoses and further investigations.

Question 7.5

A 48-year-old man presents with constitutional symptoms and acute tonsillitis. He undergoes tonsillectomy, complicated by postoperative bleeding necessitating reintubation and a return to theatre. The full blood count, blood picture and coagulation profile were examined following surgery was as follows:

Hb	84 g/L	(115–160)
WBC	35.2 × 10⁹/L	(3.5–11.0)
Platelets	52 × 10⁹/L	(140–400)
INR	2.4	(0.9–1.3)
APTT	56 s	(25–38)
Fibrinogen	0.6 g/L	(1.5–4.0)
D-Dimer	2.1	(<0.2)

Film: 40% hypergranular promyelocytes with Auer rods. Peroxidase stain positive. Schistocytes present. Platelet count consistent with film.

A What is the likely diagnosis and explanation for this patient's postoperative haemorrhage?

Question 7.6

Prothrombin ratio	1.0 INR	(0.8–1.2)
APTT	48 s	(24–39)
Platelets	230 × 10⁹/L	(150–450)
Fibrinogen	2.6 g/L	(1.5–4)
FDPs	<10 mg/L	(0–10)
Bleeding time	14 min	(0–10)

A Suggest two differential diagnoses for the above coagulation profile.

Question 7.7

A 25-year-old man with known HIV infection presents to the Emergency Department with headache, obtundation and temperature 38.1°C. Petechiae are noted over his trunk. He proceeds to a generalized seizure. Biochemical and haematological profiles are as follows:

Na$^+$	138 mmol/L	(135–145)
K$^+$	4.2 mmol/L	(3.2–4.5)
Cl$^-$	98 mmol/L	(100–110)
HCO$_3$$^-$	23 mmol/L	(22–33)
Urea	18 mmol/L	(3.0–8.0)
Creatinine	0.28 mmol/L	(0.07–0.12)
Albumin	38 g/L	(33–47)
Total bilirubin	5 umol/L	(<20)
AST	120 U/L	(<40)
ALT	78 U/L	(<45)
LDH	689 U/L	(110–250)
Hb	89 g/L	(115–160)
Platelets	25 × 10^9/L	(140–400)
INR	1.2	
APTT	36 s	(25–38)
Fibrinogen	2.5 g/L	(1.5–4.0)
Direct Coombs'	Negative	

Film: Schistocytes.

A What is the likely diagnosis?

Question 7.8

List four differential diagnoses for the coagulation profile shown below.

Prothrombin ratio INR	1.1	(0.8–1.2)
APTT	36 s	(24–39)
Platelets	240 × 10^9/L	(150–450)
Bleeding time	13 min	(2–8)
Fibrinogen	2.8 g/L	(1.5–4.0)
FDPs	<10 mg/L	(0–10)

Question 7.9

A 2-year-old child is floppy and unresponsive.

Prothrombin time	>200 s	(12–17)
APTT	>200 s	(24–39)
Fibrinogen	0.1 g/L	(1.5–4)
Platelets	270 × 10^9/L	(150–450)

A What is the likely diagnosis?

Question 7.1: Answer

A The main abnormality is prolongation of PT and INR. Both of these can be prolonged in vitamin K deficiency, in the presence of oral anticoagulants, in liver disease and in DIC. In this case there is evidence of vitamin K deficiency or warfarin therapy in view of the normal Echis time but prolonged prothrombin time.

Vitamin K causes γ carboxylation of the terminal glutamyl peptides of factors II, V, VII and X, which then combine with calcium and tissue phospholipid to activate the clotting cascade. In vitamin K deficiency or warfarin therapy, although adequate levels of these factors are produced, they are not activated by carboxylation. Hence the prothrombin time and the INR are prolonged. Venom from the snake *Echis multisquamatus* activates prothrombin without requiring vitamin K. Hence Echis time will be normal in vitamin K deficiency or in the presence of warfarin but will be prolonged in conditions where factor concentrations are reduced, as in liver disease.

Artefactual prolongation of PT may result from improper sample collection and in patients with increased haematocrits (>55%).

Question 7.2: Answer

A The pattern of results is consistent with liver dysfunction, which is possibly secondary to sepsis. There is no evidence of vitamin K deficiency or anticoagulant-induced coagulopathy, as the Echis time is prolonged.

Question 7.3: Answer

A Postcardiopulmonary bypass haemorrhage always raises the possibility of heparin-related anticoagulation. However, in this instance there is no evidence of heparin-related anticoagulation given a normal thrombin clotting time (TCT). A consumptive or dilutional coagulopathy has occurred and requires correction with platelets and fresh frozen plasma or cryoprecipitate.

TCT tests the conversion of fibrinogen to fibrin. It is performed by measuring the clotting time after the addition of excess thrombin to undiluted plasma. The test may be prolonged in the presence of hypofibrinogenaemia, fibrin degradation products (FDPs) and heparin.

Question 7.4: Answer

A Prolongation of the APTT suggests a deficiency (hereditary or acquired) of one of the clotting factors or the presence of an inhibitor. The former is diagnosed by mixing equal volumes of patient's plasma and pooled normal plasma and repeating the test. Correction of APTT to normal suggests the presence of a deficiency. Failure of the APTT to correct with 50% normal plasma (as in this case) implies a circulating inhibitor of coagulation, e.g. lupus anticoagulant. These circulating inhibitors of coagulation are seen in patients with collagen vascular disease and cancer. Follow-up investigation for anticardiolipin antibodies and an autoantibody screen would be appropriate.

Although patients with cancer are prophylactically commenced on low molecular weight heparins (LMWH) for antithrombotic prophylaxis, LMWH produce minimal perturbation in APTT. LMWH are monitored using anti-Xa activity.

Question 7.5: Answer

A The patient has typical features of promyelocytic leukaemia, M3 variant AML (FAB classification). This condition is strongly associated with disseminated intravascular coagulation (present in this patient as evidenced by prolonged PT and APTT, thrombocytopenia, the presence of D-dimers and peripheral smear showing schistocytes). The DIC can be life-threatening, particularly upon induction of chemotherapy and the subsequent release of procoagulants, unless all-*trans*-retinoic acid (ATRA) is administered to differentiate tumour cells. Heparin therapy has been shown to be effective. ATRA is also associated with a syndrome of leukocytosis, fever, dyspnoea, pleural and pericardial effusions and hypotension.

Question 7.6: Answer

A The principal coagulation abnormalities are a prolonged APTT and bleeding time (with normal platelets). The two differential diagnoses for this combination of coagulation abnormalities are:

1. von Willebrand's disease. (The diagnosis can be confirmed by the demonstration of impaired ristocetin-induced platelet aggregation and reduced factor VIII activity).

2. Combination of aspirin and heparin therapy in patients with myocardial ischaemia. (Aspirin prolongs bleeding time by blocking the synthesis of thromboxane A_2. The effect lasts for 4–7 days).

Other differentials include:

1. Postcardiopulmonary bypass (CPB), although frequently the platelet count may be low. The prolongation of bleeding time is related to the duration of CPB. CPB has been shown to reduce platelet aggregation to ristocetin and other agonists.

2. Post haemodialysis for an uraemic patient (prolonged APTT from heparin use and prolonged BT from uraemia).

Question 7.7: Answer

A Thrombotic thrombocytopenic purpura. The patient has a microangiopathic haemolytic anaemia with normal coagulation parameters, severe thrombocytopenia and evidence of renal dysfunction. Focal neurologic dysfunction is also characteristic. The presence of fragmented red cells, a sine qua non of this disorder, is characterized by schistocytes or helmet cells. Rarely biopsy of skin, muscle, gingiva, lymph node or bone marrow may be required to demonstrate typical microaneurysms and fibrin deposits. Antinuclear antibody is positive in 20% of patients. The condition is associated with HIV, pregnancy, connective tissue disorders, malignancy, and the use of drugs such as ciclosporin, quinine, ticlopidine and clopidogrel.

Whereas fever, neurological symptoms and purpura suggest an intracranial infection such as meningitis or meningococcaemia, the presence of severe renal dysfunction at presentation is unlikely.

Question 7.8: Answers

The results reveal a prolonged bleeding time in the presence of a normal platelet count, suggesting a qualitative disorder of platelet function. The most likely causes in the intensive care setting include:

- Uraemia
- Use of β–lactam antibiotics
- Use of non-steroidal anti-inflammatory drugs
- Post cardiopulmonary bypass.

The platelet dysfunction in uraemia improves with dialysis and the administration of DDAVP (desmopressin). DDAVP is administered at a dose of 0.3 µg/kg (maximum dose 20 µg) over 30 minutes. The improvement in bleeding time is apparent within 30–60 minutes of administration. However, the duration of its effect lasts only 4 hours. There are reports that increasing the haematocrit improves the platelet dysfunction in uraemia.

β-Lactam antibiotic-related platelet dysfunction is seen with most of the penicillins. The frequency of abnormal platelet function is greater with carbenicillin, penicillin G and ticarcillin than with piperacillin. The effect on platelets is maximal in the first three days after administration and lasts for many days after cessation of therapy. The treatment for bleeding associated with antibiotic-induced platelet dysfunction is cessation of the drug.

The other two conditions have been discussed in a previous section.

Question 7.9: Answer

A The likely diagnosis is coagulopathy from snake bite. The results reveal a grossly elevated PT and APTT together with very low fibrinogen. These are suggestive of marked fibrinolysis. The presence of normal platelets would argue against a DIC. Such extensive defibrination is characteristic of envenomation from snake bite. The effect of the snake venom is to initiate thrombin-like activity, cleaving fibrinopeptide A from fibrinogen and causing fibrinogenolysis. Snake venom has also been known to cause thrombocytopenia, activation of factors X and V and endothelial damage.

Although thrombolytic therapy can produce severe fibrinolysis, such a degree of defibrination is uncommon.

Further reading

Barbui T, Falanga A Disseminated intravascular coagulation in acute leukemia. Semin Thromb Hemost 2001; 27:593–604

Bennett CL, Connors JM, Carwile JM et al. Thrombotic thrombocytopenic purpura associated with clopidogrel. N Engl J Med 2000; 342:1773–1777

Bennett CL, Davidson CJ, Raisch DW, Weinberg PD, Bennett RH, Feldman MD Thrombotic thrombocytopenic purpura associated with ticlopidine in the setting of coronary artery stents and stroke prevention. Arch Intern Med 1999; 159:2524–2528

Gallanakis D Thrombin time. In: Beutler E, Lichtman M, Coller B, Kipps T, eds. Williams Hematology. New York: McGraw-Hill, 1995:L91–L93

George J, El-Harake M Thrombocytopoenia due to enhanced platelet destruction by non-immunological mechanisms. In: Beutler E, Lichtman M, Coller B, Kipps T, eds. Williams Hematology. New York: McGraw-Hill, 1995:1290–1315

Gralnick H, Ginsburg D von Willebrand disease. In: Beutler E, Lichtman M, Coller B, Kipps T, eds. Williams Hematology. New York: McGraw-Hill, 1995:1458–1485

Miletich J Prothrombin time. In: Beutler E, Lichtman M, Coller B, Kipps T, eds. Williams Hematology. New York: McGraw-Hill, 1995:L82–L84

Petrovan R, Rapaport S, Le D A novel clotting assay for quantitation of plasma prothrombin (factor II) using Echis multisquamatus venom. Am J Clin Pathol 1999; 112:705–711

Seligsohn U Disseminated intravascular coagulation. In: Beutler E, Lichtman M, Coller B, Kipps T, eds. Williams Hematology. New York: McGraw-Hill, 1995:1507

Shattil S, Bennett J Acquired qualitative platelet disorders due to diseases, drugs and foods. In: Beutler E, Lichtman M, Coller B, Kipps T, eds. Williams Hematology. New York: McGraw-Hill, 1995:1386–1400

8

Haematology

Question 8.1

A 35-year-old woman is recovering from multiple organ dysfunction syndrome subsequent to intra-abdominal sepsis from a perforated appendix. Full blood count and iron studies are as follows:

Hb	95 g/L	(120–160)
WBC	10.0×10^9/L	(4.0–10.5)
Platelets	230×10^9/L	(150–400)
PCV	0.28	(0.35– 0.49)
RBC	3.7×10^{12}/L	(4.3–5.7)
MCV	81 fL	(83–98)
MCH	23.6 pg	(28.0–33.0)
MCHC	322 g/L	(330–360)
Serum iron	4 µmol/L	(10–32)
Serum ferritin	190 µg/L	(15–200)
Serum transferrin	1.1 g/L	(1.9–3.0)
Saturation	15%	(15–54)

A What is the most likely cause of her anaemia?

Question 8.2

An 18-year-old male presents with abdominal pain and dizziness 24 hours after a football match. He has a diffusely tender abdomen. The following is his full blood count:

Hb	84 g/L	(130–175)
WBC	8.3×10^9/L	(4.0–11.0)
Platelets	240×10^9/L	(150–450)
Reticulocytes	180×10^9/L	(10–80)
Neutrophils	5.8×10^9/L	(1.8–7.5)
Lymphocytes	1.5×10^9/L	(1.5–4.0)
Monocytes	0.4×10^9/L	(0.2–0.8)
Eosinophils	0.6×10^9/L	(0.0–0.4)
Haematocrit	0.25	(0.4–0.52)
MCV	88.4 fL	(82–98)
MCH	30.2 pg	(27.0–34.0)
MCHC	341 g/L	(310–360)

A What is the most likely cause of the abnormalities?

Question 8.3

The patient in the preceding question requires a laparotomy. On postoperative day 5 coagulation studies and full blood count are as follows:

Prothrombin ratio	0.9 INR	(0.8–1.2)
APTT	33 s	(24–39)
Fibrinogen	6.1 g/L	(1.5–4.0)
Hb	104 g/L	(130–175)
WBC	15.7×10^9/L	(4.0–11.0)
Platelets	960×10^9/L	(150–450)
Reticulocytes	89×10^9/L	(10–80)
Neutrophils	13.7×10^9/L	(1.8–7.5)
Lymphocytes	2.0×10^9/L	(1.5–4.0)

Comment: Moderate anisocytosis. Slight poikilocytosis. Occasional target cells. Howell–Jolly bodies present.

A Why is the fibrinogen elevated?

B What is the likely explanation for the thrombocytosis?

Question 8.4

A 25-year-old woman is admitted to ICU with 60% surface burns and treated along standard lines. On day 3 she is normotensive and well perfused, with a core temperature of 38°C. Her urine output and renal biochemistry are normal, and she has a normal conscious state. Her full blood count shows the following abnormality:

Hb	154 g/L	(130–175)
WBC	1.8×10^9/L	(4.0–11.0)
Platelets	180×10^9/L	(150–450)
Neutrophils	0.3×10^9/L	(1.8–7.5)
Lymphocytes	1.1×10^9/L	(1.5–4.0)
Monocytes	0.4×10^9/L	(0.2–0.8)
Haematocrit	0.46	(0.4–0.52)

A What is the likely diagnosis?

B What is the likely underlying cause?

C What should be done?

Question 8.5

A 50-year–old man has been in a medical ward for 3 days with bronchopneumonia. You are asked to review him because of new episodes of desaturation on pulse oximetry, despite an improved chest X-ray. He is combative, disorientated in time and place, and calling out inappropriately. He appears to be experiencing visual and auditory hallucinations. There is generalized mild hyperreflexia. His full blood count is as follows:

Hb	152 g/L	(130–175)
WBC	15.6×10^9/L	(4.0–11.0)
Platelets	158×10^9/L	(150–450)
Neutrophils	13.8×10^9/L	(1.8–7.5)
Lymphocytes	1.5×10^9/L	(1.5–4.0)
Monocytes	0.3×10^9/L	(0.2–0.8)
Haematocrit	0.46	(0.4–0.52)
MCV	106 fL	(82–98)
MCH	35 pg	(27.0–34.0)
MCHC	330 g/L	(310–360)

A What is the *most likely* explanation for the clinical and haematological picture?

B Give reasons.

C What is the likely reason for the desaturation?

Question 8.6

A 16-year-old girl is admitted with status asthmaticus after an upper respiratory tract infection. The following is her full blood count on arrival:

Hb	154 g/L	(130–175)
WBC	4.9×10^9/L	(4.0–11.0)
Platelets	277×10^9/L	(150–450)
Neutrophils	4.3×10^9/L	(1.8–7.5)
Lymphocytes	0.4×10^9/L	(1.5–4.0)
Monocytes	0.2×10^9/L	(0.2–0.8)
Haematocrit	0.46	(0.4–0.52)
MCV	84 fL	(82–98)
MCH	28.3 pg	(27.0–34.0)
MCHC	336 g/L	(310–360)

A What is the likely explanation for the lymphopenia?

B What other types of critical illness can be associated with lymphopenia?

Question 8.7

A 25-year-old male with type 1 diabetes mellitus presents with severe diabetic ketoacidosis. He has epigastric pain and has been vomiting. He is alert, not shocked, and has a non-tender abdomen. The following is his full blood count on admission:

Hb	190 g/L	(130–175)
WBC	28 × 10⁹/L	(4.0–11.0)
Platelets	425 × 10⁹/L	(150–450)
Neutrophils	27 × 10⁹/L	(1.8–7.5)
Lymphocytes	0.2 × 10⁹/L	(1.5–4.0)
Monocytes	0.2 × 10⁹/L	(0.2–0.8)
Metamyelocytes	occ	
Myelocytes	occ	
Red cell count	6.9 × 10¹²/L	(4.0–5.5)
Haematocrit	0.62	(0.4–0.52)
MCV	90 fl	(82–98)
MCH	28.0 pg	(27.0–34.0)
MCHC	306 g/L	(310–360)

Neutrophils show left shift.

A What is the likely cause of the polycythaemia?

B What is the most likely cause of the abnormal neutrophil and lymphocyte counts?

Question 8.8

A 38-year-old woman with rheumatic valvular disease and a mitral valve prosthesis presents with breathlessness and a new pansystolic murmur on auscultation at the apex.

Hb	121 g/L	(115–160)
RCC	4.21×10^{12}/L	(3.8–5.2)
Reticulocytes	160×10^9/L	(10–100)
Haptoglobin	0 g/L	(0.35–2.20)
Direct Coombs'	Negative	
Heinz bodies	0%	

A Suggest a likely cause of this woman's presentation and why?

B Suggest two treatment measures.

Question 8.1: Answer

A Anaemia of chronic disease.

The pattern of anaemia with mild microcytosis, normochromia, absent reticulocyte response, low serum iron, transferrin and % saturation with normal ferritin is most consistent with this diagnosis. Lack of an increase in serum transferrin receptor concentration (see below) and the absence of a haemoglobin increment in response to oral iron are confirmatory. Occasionally bone marrow biopsy is necessary to confirm the presence of adequate iron stores. Anaemia of chronic disease occurs in the setting of infections and inflammation (as in this case), and also in neoplasia.

The transferrin receptor, a fragment of the cellular receptor, circulates in the plasma bound to transferrin. Serum concentrations reflect the cellular mass of these receptors. Receptor synthesis is increased in iron deficiency anaemia, but not in the anaemia of chronic disease. The most important clinical use of the serum transferrin receptor is in determining the presence of iron-deficient erythropoiesis (that is, identifying iron deficiency anemia, whether it occurs alone or in the presence of the anaemia of chronic disease).

Question 8.2: Answer

A Acute blood loss.

There is a normochromic normocytic anaemia with a reticulocytosis, which in this setting is most likely due to acute blood loss. In other clinical settings low-grade haemolysis is also a possibility. Reticulocytosis may be detected within 6–12 hours after the onset of haemorrhage and appears to be induced by erythropoietin.

Question 8.3: Answers

A Acute-phase response.

B Post splenectomy combined with acute-phase response. The absence of splenic function can be inferred from certain haematological changes. These include:

(a) Leukocytosis

(b) Thrombocytosis

(c) Howell–Jolly bodies (these are nuclear fragments within red cells, which are normally removed in the spleen. Only 1 out of 100–1000 red cells is affected)

(d) Pitted red cells and target cells.

Question 8.4: Answers

A Early post-burn leukopenia (EPBL).

B The cause is unknown, but silver sulfadiazine treatment may be contributory. Overwhelming sepsis is unlikely in view of the clinical findings and the absence of toxic granulation.

C Most practitioners would cease the silver sulfadiazine and use an alternative topical agent (e.g. mafenide acetate). Rapid resolution should be expected – the condition is usually self-limiting (even with continuation of silver sulfadiazine). If the neutropenia fails to resolve within 72 hours, a bone marrow biopsy should be performed. Both maturation arrest and hypercellularity have been described in EPBL. Other causes of sudden neutropenia, such as acute leukaemia, and drugs such as cimetidine need to be excluded. GCSF treatment may be required.

Question 8.5: Answers

A Acute alcohol withdrawal.

B Acute alcohol withdrawal often manifests within 48 hours of stopping drinking. There is a neutrophilia in keeping with a response to pulmonary infection. There is a macrocytosis without anaemia. The likely cause of the macrocytosis in this case is alcoholism. The macrocytosis of alcoholism is present in 80–90% of chronic alcoholics, unrelated to liver disease or vitamin deficiency. The MCV returns to normal after 2–4 months of abstinence.

Other causes of macrocytosis include chronic liver disease, hypothyroidism, cytotoxic agents and the reticulocytosis of low-grade haemolysis. Cobalamin and folate deficiency cause megaloblastic anaemia with more severe peripheral macrocytosis, as do folate antagonists. Nevertheless, serum B_{12} and red cell folate levels should be checked.

C Removal of supplemental oxygen by a combative and restless patient. Hypoxaemia is a rare cause of confusion and combativeness in critical illness. The reverse scenario is, however, quite common. Here confusion and combativeness exacerbate hypoxaemia because the patient constantly removes all sources of supplemental oxygen, such as masks and nasal cannulae.

Question 8.6: Answers

A Likely causes include a simple stress response, the preceding viral infection, or prior corticosteroid administration.

B Severe sepsis, autoimmune diseases such as systemic lupus erythematosis, tuberculosis, brucellosis, histoplasmosis, HIV infection, other viral infections such as cytomegalovirus, cytotoxic drugs, radiation.

Question 8.7: Answers

A Relative polycythaemia (normal red cell mass, but reduced plasma volume) due to dehydration.

B Neutrophilia with left shift (immature forms) is a common stress response in severe diabetic ketoacidosis. Major non-leukaemic elevations in neutrophil counts, with the appearance of immature forms, can be seen in severe infection (often as an overshoot after transient neutropenia) or in other stressful conditions such as severe shock. If the neutrophil count exceeds $50 \times 10^9/L$, these are known as leukaemoid reactions. Underlying infection as a cause of neutrophilia is suggested by toxic granulation, Döhle bodies or cytoplasmic vacuoles (not seen in this case). The lymphopenia is also probably stress related.

Question 8.8: Answers

A Paravalvular mitral prosthetic leak with pulmonary oedema. There is evidence of mechanical haemolysis. Traumatic haemolysis is more common with aortic (approximately 10%) than with mitral prosthesis, because of the higher pressure gradients across the aortic valve. The incidence of paravalvular haemolysis is greater with smaller valves, mechanical prostheses, and in the presence of a paravalvular leak. Heinz bodies are a feature of drug-induced oxidant haemolysis, whereas Coombs' tests become positive with immune haemolysis.

B Erythropoiesis should be optimized by folate and iron supplements. Valve replacement should be considered if haemolysis is severe or significant cardiac failure occurs.

Further reading

Babior B, Bunn HM-Hp- Megaloblastic anemias. In: Isselbacher K, Braunwald E, Wilson J, Martin J, Fauci A, Kasper D, eds. Harrison's principles of internal medicine, 13th edn. New York: McGraw-Hill, 1994; 1726–1732

Curnutte J, Coates T Disorderes of phagocyte function and number. In: Hoffman R, Benz E, Shattil S et al., eds. Hematology. Basic principles and practice. New York: Churchill Livingstone, 2000; 720–762

Fuller F, Engler P Leukopenia in non-septic burn patients receiving topical 1% silver sulfadiazine cream therapy: A survey. J Burn Care Rehab 1988; 9:606–609

Rosenthal D Hematological manifestations of infectious disease. In: Hoffman R, Benz E, Shattil S et al., eds. Hematology. Basic principles and practice, 3rd edn. New York: Churchill Livingstone, 2000; 2420–2430

Rosse W, Bunn H Hemolytic anemias and acute blood loss. In: Fauci A et al., eds. Harrison's principles of internal medicine, 14th edn. New York: McGraw–Hill, 1998; 668

Sears D Anaemia of chronic disease. Med Clin North Am 1992; 76:567–579

Thrasher A, Segal A Leucocytes in health and disease. In: Weatherall D, Ledingham J, Warrell D, eds. Oxford textbook of medicine. Oxford: Oxford University Press, 1996; 3555–3561

9

Intoxications

Question 9.1

A 28-year-old patient presents to the emergency department in coma. He is noted to have rapid deep respirations. There are no other significant findings on clinical examination.

Initial test results are as follows:

CT brain: No abnormality detected		
CSF: No abnormality detected		
FiO$_2$	0.21	
pH	7.10	
PCO$_2$	14 mmHg	
PO$_2$	112 mmHg	
Sodium	131 mmol/L	(135–145)
Potassium	3 mmol/L	(3.2–4.5)
Glucose	14 mmol/L	(3–7.8)
Urea	10 mmol/L	(3–8)
Creatinine	0.07 mmol/L	(0.07–0.12)
Bicarbonate	16 mmol/L	(22–33)
Chloride	94 mmol/L	(100–110)
Serum osmolality (meas)	324 mosm/Kg	(280–290)
Ionized calcium	1.2 mmol/L	(1.1–1.3)

24 hours later he is noted to have fixed dilated pupils.

A What biochemical pathology is evident?

B Suggest a likely diagnosis.

Question 9.2

A previously well 45-year-old farmer was admitted to the intensive care unit with abdominal pain, nausea and vomiting. He was due in court the next day. Apart from pharyngeal ulceration, physical examination was normal.

Investigations were as follows:

FBC		
Hb	149 gL	(120–160)
WBC	11×10^9/L	(4.0–10.5)
Platelets	221×10^9/L	(150–400)

ABG		
FiO_2	0.5	
pH	7.46	
PCO_2	32 mmHg	
PO_2	84 mmHg	

Sodium	37 mmol/L	(135–145)
Potassium	4.7 mmol/L	(3.2–4.5)
Urea	10.7 mmol/L	(3.0–8.0)
Creat	0.13 mmol/L	(0.07–0.12)
Glucose	6.4 mmol/L	(3.0–7.8)
Coags NAD		

A What is the likely diagnosis?

B Suggest two tests you would use to confirm the diagnosis.

C List two principles of management.

Question 9.3

A previously well 28-year-old man collapsed in the Arrivals Lounge of Brisbane International Airport. He had seizures in the ambulance en route to the hospital. On arrival at the Accident and Emergency department the following findings were evident:

GCS 3		
Temp 40.1°C		
HR 140/min, sinus tachycardia		
BP 210/120		
Pupils 8 mm, sluggishly reactive		
Perforated nasal septum +		
ECG: ST depression and T wave inversion in V1–V3		
Sodium	146 mmol/L	(135–145)
Potassium	4.5 mmol/L	(3.2–4.5)
Urea	8.7 mmol/L	(3.0–8.0)
Creat	0.21 mmol/L	(0.07–0.12)
CK	14 000 U/L	(50–150)

A Suggest a likely diagnosis.

B Suggest one diagnostic test.

Question 9.4

A 70-year-old woman with long-standing stable rheumatoid arthritis was admitted to the intensive care unit with breathlessness. Investigations on admission were as follows:

Hb	54 g/L	(120–160)
WBC	2.1×10^9/L	(4.0–10.5)
Platelets	74×10^9/L	(150–400)
MCV	107 fL	(83–98)

A Suggest two causes of breathlessness in this patient.

B What is the likely cause of the blood picture?

C How will you treat the underlying cause of her anaemia?

Question 9.5

A 34-year-old man was admitted to ICU after having been found unconscious at home by his mother. There was a history of head injury and post-traumatic epilepsy.

O/E GCS 3
Temp 35.5°C
No neck stiffness
Pupils midsized and reactive
Tense bullous lesions were found over his fingers, elbows and ankles.
CT brain scan: NAD
CSF studies: Normal.

A Suggest a likely diagnosis.

B Outline three principles of management.

Question 9.1: Answers

A The biochemistry reveals:

- A high anion gap (AG = 21) metabolic acidosis

- A raised osmolar gap (36)

B The clinical picture and a history of a normal CT scan and CSF studies suggest a drug overdose. This in conjunction with the biochemical picture indicates an alcohol ingestion (raised osmolar gap and anion gap). The subsequent development of fixed dilated pupils suggests methanol overdose. (The presence of normal ionized calcium together with the rest of the clinical picture argues against ethylene glycol ingestion. For completeness, plasma β-hydroxybutyrate should be measured to exclude ketoacidosis).

Following ingestion methanol toxicity usually manifests within 30 hours (range 40 min–72 h) of ingestion. The clinical features are largely confined to the CNS, ocular and gastrointestinal systems. Visual symptoms and signs are related to concentrations of formic acid, a metabolite of methanol metabolism. Fundoscopy may show disc hyperaemia and papilloedema.

Question 9.2: Answers

A The likely diagnosis is paraquat poisoning. This is based on the following:

- Easy access to paraquat, given the patient's occupation

- Presence of pharyngeal ulceration

- Respiratory and renal dysfunction.

- The history of imminent court appearance may have precipitated the attempted suicide.

B

- Plasma paraquat assay, useful for confirmation of diagnosis and prognosis

- Sodium dithionite test on a urine specimen. If the urine colour changes to blue on addition of dithionite, it confirms paraquat exposure. This provides a rapid qualitative screen for paraquat exposure.

C Two important principles of management include:

- Prevention of systemic absorption using enteric Fuller's earth or activated charcoal

- Monitoring and therapy of ARDS. Avoid unnecessary exposure to high FiO_2. Charcoal haemoperfusion has not been demonstrated to improve mortality.

Question 9.3: Answers

A The clinical scenario is highly suggestive of cocaine intoxication. The differential diagnosis should include catecholaminergic states such as phaeochromocytoma, thyrotoxicosis, and poisonings such as amphetamine, theophyllines, and phencyclidine. The elevated serum CK and creatinine indicate significant rhabdomyolysis.

B A urinary screen for cocaine metabolites.

Question 9.4: Answers

A Two likely causes of breathlessness include:

• Rheumatoid lung

• Anaemia.

With a history of immunosuppression, opportunistic infections such as pneumocystis pneumonia should also be considered.

B The most likely cause of her anaemia is methotrexate-induced pancytopenia from folate antagonism.

C Folinic acid rescue.

Question 9.5: Answers

A The likely diagnosis is barbiturate overdose, because of:

• The circumstantial nature of the coma

• The likelihood of the patient being on long-term anticonvulsants

• Findings of tense bullae (although not specific for barbiturate overdose, these are seen in about 6% of cases)

• Normal CT and CSF studies.

B After confirmation of the diagnosis using serum barbiturate levels, three important principles of management include:

• Support of airway, breathing and circulation

• Multiple dose charcoal lavage to facilitate gastrointestinal clearance

• Alkaline diuresis may be helpful. Haemoperfusion has been shown to be effective.

Further reading

Aaron C, Burke M, Restuccia M, Nichols C, Scmidt E. Sedative-hypnotic poisoning. In: Rippe J, Irwin R, Fink M, Cerra F, editors. Intensive Care Medicine. Boston: Little Brown and Company, 1996:1693-1701

Chiang W, Wang R. Pesticide poisoning. In: Rippe J, Irwin R, Fink M, Cerra F, eds. Intensive Care Medicine. Boston: Little Brown and Company, 1996:1663-1685

Ford M Alcohols and glycols. In: Rippe J, Irwin R, Fink M, Cerra F, eds. Intensive Care Medicine. Boston: Little Brown and Company, 1996:1506–1520

Renzi F Cocaine poisoning. In: Rippe J, Irwin R, Fink M, Cerra F, eds. Intensive Care Medicine. Boston: Little Brown and Company, 1996:1553-1557

10.

Radiology

Question 10.1

This 35-year-old woman was admitted with circulatory shock and respiratory failure. There is a past history of liver disease.

A Comment on the chest X-ray findings.

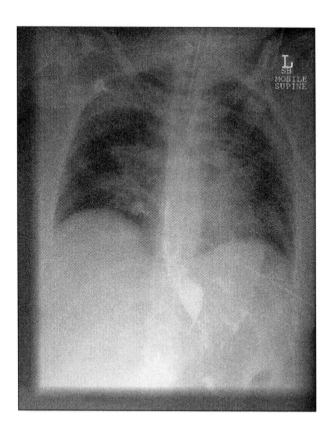

Question 10.2

This is the chest X-Ray of a 77-year-old woman admitted with fever and shock.

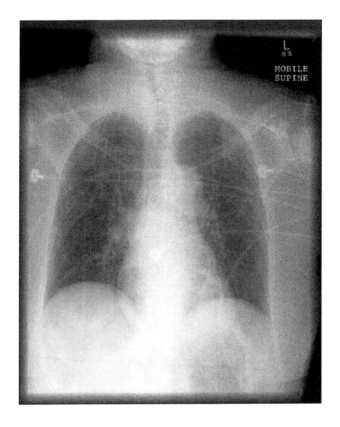

A What is the principal abnormality on the chest X-Ray ?

B List two investigations you would perform to identify the source of sepsis ?

Question 10.3

Examine the chest X-ray of the patient intubated and ventilated for severe asthma.

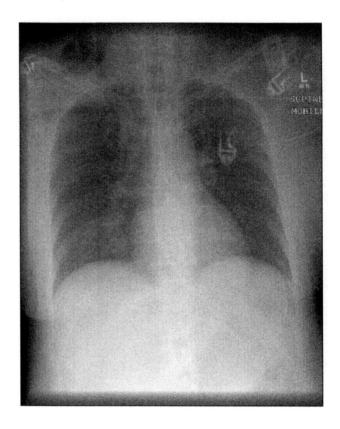

A What are the abnormalities?

B Describe the pathogenesis of the abnormalities.

Question 10.4

A Describe the abnormalities on the chest X-Ray.

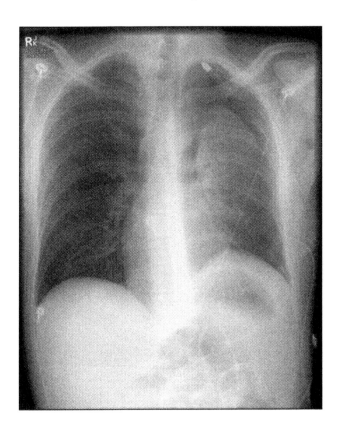

Question 10.5

This is the CT scan of a patient after a head injury.

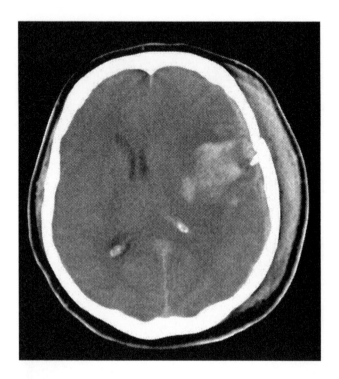

A List four abnormal findings.

Question 10.1: Answer

A The findings on the chest X-ray include:

- Bilateral alveolar infiltrates in the middle and lower zones

- There is also a radio-opaque dye seen in the lower oesophagus and stomach. This is glue used to obliterate oesophageal and gastric varices

- An endotracheal tube and a right internal jugular central venous line are in place.

This patient had a massive haematemesis, resulting in circulatory shock and aspiration pneumonia.

Question 10.2: Answers

A The abnormality seen on the chest X-Ray is the presence of a ventriculoperitoneal shunt.

B The two investigations will include:

- Tapping the VP shunt for CSF cell count, microbiology and biochemistry

- Blood culture and sensitivity

Question 10.3: Answers

A The abnormalities include subcutaneous emphysema in the neck bilaterally, gas in the strap muscles of the neck and mediastinal emphysema, all of which are consistent with pulmonary barotrauma. There is incipient right bronchial intubation.

Clinical manifestations of barotrauma include pulmonary interstitial emphysema, pneumothorax, subcutaneous emphysema, pneumoperitoneum, tension lung cysts, subpleural air cysts and venous air embolization.

B The first stage in the development of barotrauma is the rupture of an alveolus. When this happens, air introduced into the pulmonary interstitium travels along the perivascular spaces into the mediastinum, resulting in a pneumomediastinum. This gas then travels along fascial planes into the neck, resulting in subcutaneous emphysema in the neck or into the retroperitoneal space. With increase in mediastinal pressure the mediastinal parietal pleura may rupture, resulting in a pneumothorax.

Question 10.4: Answer

A The chest X-Ray reveals the following:

- A left-sided pneumothorax with an intercostal catheter in situ

- Surgical clips in the incision line of a left thoracotomy

- Evidence of subcutaneous air in the left side of the neck

- The elevated left hemidiaphragm and attenuation of the left main bronchus indicates that sputum plugging rather than ongoing air leak is the main cause of the loss of left lung volume.

Question 10.5: Answers

A

- Fracture of left parietal bone and an associated scalp haematoma

- Acute left parietal subdural haematoma

- Large acute left parietal intracerebral haematoma

- Midline shift to the right.

Glossary

A-a gradient	Alveolar-arterial gradient
ALP	Alkaline phosphatase
CI	Cardiac index
CK	Creatinine kinase
CO	Cardiac output
Coags	Coagulation screen
CVP	Central venous pressure
FiO_2	Fraction of inspired oxygen concentration
GGT	Gamma glutamyl transpeptidase
Hb/Hgb	Haemoglobin
HCO_3^-	Bicarbonate
HR	Heart rate
MAP	Mean arterial pressure
MCV	Mean corpuscular volume
NAD	No abnormality detected
PAO_2	Partial pressure of oxygen in the alveolus
PAOP	Pulmonary artery occlusion pressure
PAP	Pulmonary artery pressure
PCO_2	Partial pressure of carbon dioxide
PO_2	Partial pressure of oxygen
PO4	Phosphate
PVR	Pulmonary vascular resistance
RA	Right atrium
RV	Right ventricle
SaO_2	Oxygen saturation of haemoglobin in the arterial blood
SIADH	Syndrome of inappropriate antidiuretic hormone secretion
SVO_2	Mixed venous oxygen saturation
SVRI	Systemic vascular resistance index
Temp	Temperature
$\dot{V}/\dot{Q}$	Ventilation-perfusion
VCO_2	Carbon dioxide production per minute
VO_2	Oxygen consumption per minute
WBC	White cell count

Index

Printed and bound by CPI Group (UK) Ltd, Croydon, CR0 4YY

03/10/2024

01040848-0018